SOLO Taxonomy in Physical Education

essential resources

Learning through movement contexts

Book 2

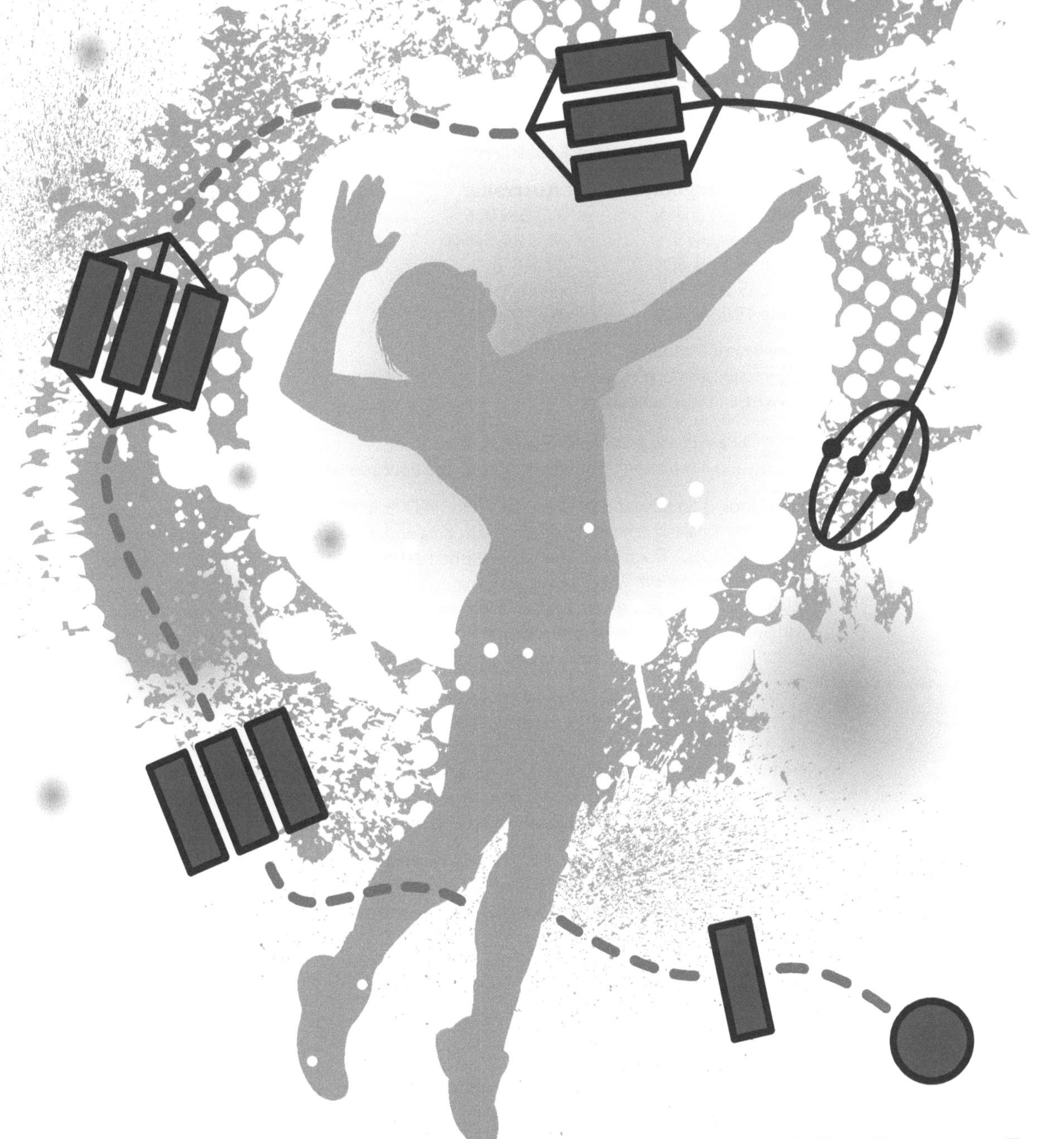

Pam Hook and Nicola Richards

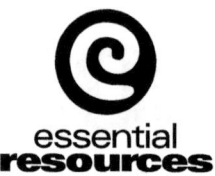

essential resources

Title:	SOLO Taxonomy in Physical Education
	Learning through movement contexts – Book 2
Authors:	Pam Hook and Nicola Richards
Editor:	Tanya Tremewan
Designer:	Diane Whitford
Book code:	5806
ISBN:	978-1-927251-37-9
Published:	2013
Publisher:	Essential Resources Educational Publishers Limited

United Kingdom:	**Australia:**	**New Zealand:**
Units 8–10 Parkside	PO Box 906	PO Box 5036
Shortgate Lane	Strawberry Hills	Invercargill
Laughton BN8 6DG	NSW 2012	
ph: 0845 3636 147	ph: 1800 005 068	ph: 0800 087 376
fax: 0845 3636 148	fax: 1800 981 213	fax: 0800 937 825

Websites: www.essentialresourcesuk.com
www.essentialresources.com.au
www.essentialresources.co.nz

Copyright: Text: © Pam Hook and Nicola Richards, 2013
Edition and illustrations: © Essential Resources Educational Publishers Limited, 2013

About the authors: Pam Hook is an educational consultant (HookED Educational Consultancy), who works with New Zealand schools to develop curricula and pedagogies for learning to learn based on SOLO Taxonomy. She has published articles on thinking, learning, e-learning and gifted education, writes curriculum material for government and business, directs Ministry of Education e-learning contracts and is co-author of two science textbooks widely used in New Zealand secondary schools. She is known for her educational blog (http://artichoke.typepad.com) and is a popular keynote speaker at conferences.

Nicola Richards has taught physical education and health in New Zealand schools for the past 18 years. She is currently teaching at St Andrew's College in Christchurch, where she has recently taken on the role of SOLO coordinator. She is passionate about creating meaningful physical education and encouraging literacy through movement contexts. As she also enjoys developing new resources for her department, Nicola leapt at the opportunity to co-author a book in an area to which she is so strongly committed.

Acknowledgements: Thanks to Professor John Biggs for his encouragement and ongoing critique of the classroom-based use of SOLO Taxonomy. We are also grateful to St Andrew's College, Christchurch, New Zealand for providing the examples of student learning outcomes used in this series.

Copyright notice:
Schools and teachers who buy this book have permission to reproduce it within their present school by photocopying, or if in digital format, by printing as well. Quantities should be reasonable for educational purposes in that school and may not be used for non-educational purposes nor supplied to anyone else. Copies made from this book, whether by photocopying or printing from a digital file, are to be included in the sampling surveys of Copyright Licensing Limited (New Zealand), Copyright Agency Limited (Australia) or Copyright Licensing Agency (United Kingdom).
For further information on your copyright obligations, visit: New Zealand: www.copyright.co.nz, Australia: www.copyright.com.au, United Kingdom: www.cla.co.uk

Contents

Introduction	4
1. SOLO strategies for movement concepts and motor skills	**5**
Using SOLO maps and rubrics	6
Using SOLO functioning knowledge rubrics	15
Using SOLO stations	19
Using a SOLO learning log	19
2. SOLO strategies for relationships with other people	**21**
Using SOLO maps and rubrics	22
Using SOLO functioning knowledge rubrics	33
3. SOLO strategies for healthy communities and environments	**40**
Using SOLO maps	41
4. Planning a student workbook with constructive alignment	**48**
Seven-step planning process	48
Example of a student workbook	54
Examples of completed SOLO maps with a fitness focus	65
Conclusion	67
References	68

Introduction

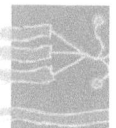

SOLO gives me structure in my thinking. It prompts me to think more deeply …

… and with SOLO rubrics I can see how to get to the next level for a physical skill.

Year 10 PE students

This *SOLO Taxonomy in Physical Education* series identifies how both the challenges and opportunities for teaching and learning in physical education (PE) can be addressed in movement contexts using SOLO Taxonomy (Biggs and Collis 1982; Biggs and Tang 2007), a simple but effective model of learning outcomes. It demonstrates the enormous potential of SOLO to build understanding in relation to each of the key competencies and PE strands of the New Zealand Curriculum:

- Book 1 introduces SOLO Taxonomy and offers ideas for introducing students to and engaging them with this model in PE settings. It also deals with the key competencies and the strand of personal health and physical development.
- Book 2 (this book) covers the other three strands – movement concepts and motor skills; relationships with other people; and healthy communities and environments. It also demonstrates how constructive alignment can be used in planning a student workbook.

Although these areas are considered separately to keep the focus of each section clear, we recognise that of course in practice the various key competencies and strands are integrated within each learning experience.

The diagram below briefly summarises the five levels of learning outcomes in SOLO Taxonomy and shows the symbol for each one. For more information, see Book 1. Please also see Book 1 for an overview of PE in the New Zealand Curriculum and of the challenges and opportunities for teaching and learning.

SOLO levels and symbols

			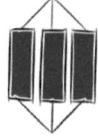	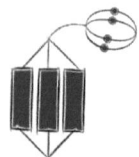
Prestructural	Unistructural	Multistructural	Relational	Extended abstract
Whakarangaranga	*Rangaranga takitahi*	*Rangaranga maha*	*Whanaungatanga*	*Waitara whānui*
Has missed point; needs help to start	Surface level – understands one aspect of task	Surface level – understands several aspects but not their relationships	Deep level – links and integrates aspects of task	Conceptual level – has new understanding from which to predict, generalise, reflect etc

Note: For a full set of HOT SOLO maps and visual self assessment rubrics, including instructions for use, see: P Hook and J Mills (2011) *SOLO Taxonomy: A guide for schools. Book 1: A common language of learning*. Invercargill: Essential Resources. For the HookED SOLO Describe++ map and self assessment rubric, see Book 1 in this *SOLO Taxonomy in Physical Education* series.

1. SOLO strategies for movement concepts and motor skills

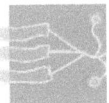
When we talked about passing and catching I could see I was still at the SOLO multistructural level and to move on I need to work on using the skills in games.

Year 10 PE student

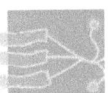
In [the movement concepts and motor skills strand,] students develop motor skills, knowledge and understandings about movement, and positive attitudes about physical activity. (Ministry of Education 2007)

The main focus of the movement concepts and motor skills strand is on development of physical literacy. However, when SOLO Taxonomy is added to the mix, students can extend their thinking and develop deeper understanding of some of the more theoretical aspects. With its rubrics, they can also be involved in feedback and feed forward. The rubrics can be self assessment tools in workbooks or teacher assessment tools, or enlarged copies can be displayed on the wall for students to use Post-it notes to identify at the start and end of the lesson where they are at. Lessons could be set up using SOLO stations to allow for differentiation of learning activities (see Section 1 of Book 1). Regardless of the pedagogy used to teach physical literacy (skills based, game sense, TGfU,[1] sport education), SOLO can deepen your students' learning outcomes.

The learning intentions in Table 1.1 were developed through constructive alignment as examples of how this strand can be explored at a deep level. It is followed by four examples of effective SOLO strategies – SOLO maps and self assessment rubrics, functioning knowledge rubrics, stations and learning logs – that can be used to explore movement concepts and motor skills in ways that develop deeper thinking in relation to the questions "why?", "to what extent?" and "what if?".

Effective SOLO strategies for movement concepts and motor skills

SOLO map

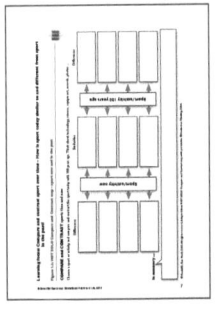

SOLO self assessment rubric

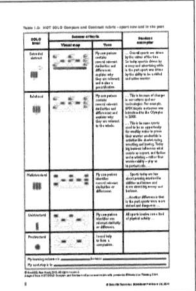

SOLO functioning knowledge rubric

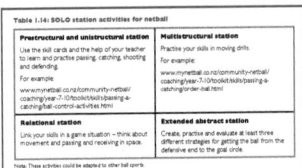

SOLO stations

SOLO learning log

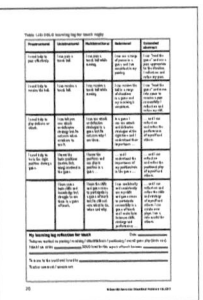

---

1 Teaching games for understanding (TGfU) teaches tactical understanding before dealing with the performance of skills. It emphasises game performance before skill performance. The why of games is taught before the how (Griffin et al 1997; Werner 1989).

Table 1.1: Possible learning intentions for exploring deep understanding of movement concepts and motor skills

Developed using constructive alignment

Unistructural and multistructural	Relational	Extended abstract
Identify skills in a game or activity. *Identify* strategies in a game or activity. *Identify* technology in activities. *Define* skill. *Define* ability. *Define* strategy, attack, defence. *Define* stages of learning. *Define* practice methods. *Define* challenge. *Define* cultural factors. *Describe* skills in a game. *Describe* the key parts of a skill or strategy. *Describe* strategies for effective participation in a game.	*Compare and contrast* different skills and strategies. *Compare and contrast* sport over time. (See Figure 1.1, Table 1.2.) *Compare and contrast* games from different cultures. *Classify* skills. *Analyse (part–whole)* skill components. *Explain* cause and effect of errors in a skill. (See Figure 1.4, Table 1.5.) *Explain* cause and effect strategies in a game. *Sequence* the stages of learning a new skill. (See Figure 1.3, Table 1.4.) *Sequence* parts of a skill. *Sequence* the history of technology in a sport. *Explain* science and technology in specific sport. *Explain* games and activities from other cultures. *Explain* how cultures can be expressed through movement.	*Evaluate* the effectiveness of skills in a game. *Evaluate* the effectiveness of strategy in a game. *Evaluate* the effectiveness of technology in a specific sport. *Create* a "perfect" skill chart. *Predict* how technology will impact on sport in the future. (See Figure 1.2, Table 1.3.) *Reflect* on own levels of skill and improvement over time. *Describe, explain and evaluate* performance.

Using SOLO maps and rubrics

The examples that follow show how SOLO maps and self assessment rubrics can be used to:
- compare and contrast sport over time (Figure 1.1 and Table 1.2)
- predict how science and technology will impact on a sport in the future (Figure 1.2 and Table 1.3)
- sequence the stages of learning a new skill (Figure 1.3 and Table 1.4)
- explain the cause and effect of errors in a skill (Figure 1.4 and Table 1.5).

Learning focus: Compare and contrast sport over time – How is sport today similar to and different from sport in the past?

Figure 1.1: HOT SOLO Compare and Contrast map – sport now and in the past

COMPARE and CONTRAST sports then and now

Choose a sport or activity and compare and contrast the sport today with 100 years ago. Think about technology, science, equipment, records, photos …

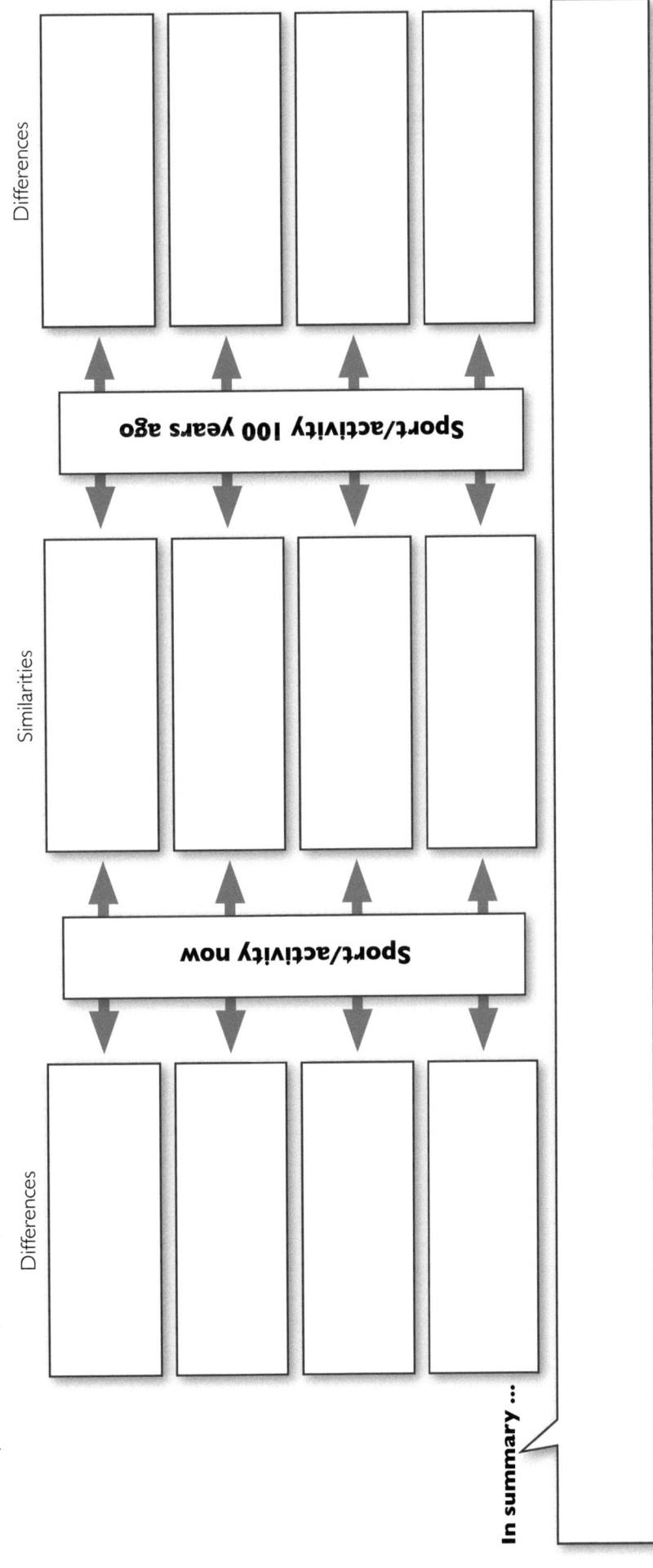

Table 1.2: HOT SOLO Compare and Contrast rubric – sport now and in the past

SOLO level	Success criteria – Visual map	Success criteria – Text	Student exemplar
Extended abstract		My comparison contains several relevant similarities and differences; explains why they are relevant; and makes a generalisation.	… Overall sports are driven by the values of the time. So today sport is driven by money and advertising while in the past sport was driven by the ability to be a skilled and active warrior.
Relational		My comparison contains several relevant similarities and differences; and explains why they are relevant to the whole.	… This is because of changes in our culture and our technologies. For example, BMX bicycle motocross was introduced to the Olympics in 2008. … This is because sports used to be an opportunity for wealthy males to prove their warrior credentials in activities like chariot racing, wrestling and boxing. Today big business influences what counts as a sport, and fashion and marketing – rather than warrior ability – play an important role. …
Multistructural		My comparison identifies several relevant similarities or differences.	… Sports today are less about proving warrior-like abilities and leisure and more about big money and business. … …Another difference is that in the past sports were more violent and dangerous. …
Unistructural		My comparison identifies one relevant similarity or difference.	All sports involve some kind of physical activity. …
Prestructural		I need help to form a comparison.	

My learning outcome is _____ because _____
My next step is to _____

© HookED, Pam Hook, 2013. All rights reserved.
Adapted from HOT SOLO Compare and Contrast self assessment rubric with permission ©Hooked on Thinking, 2004.

Learning focus: Predict how science and technology could impact on a sport in the future

Figure 1.2: **HOT SOLO Predict map** – future impact of science technology on sport

PREDICT how science and technology will impact on a specific sport in the future

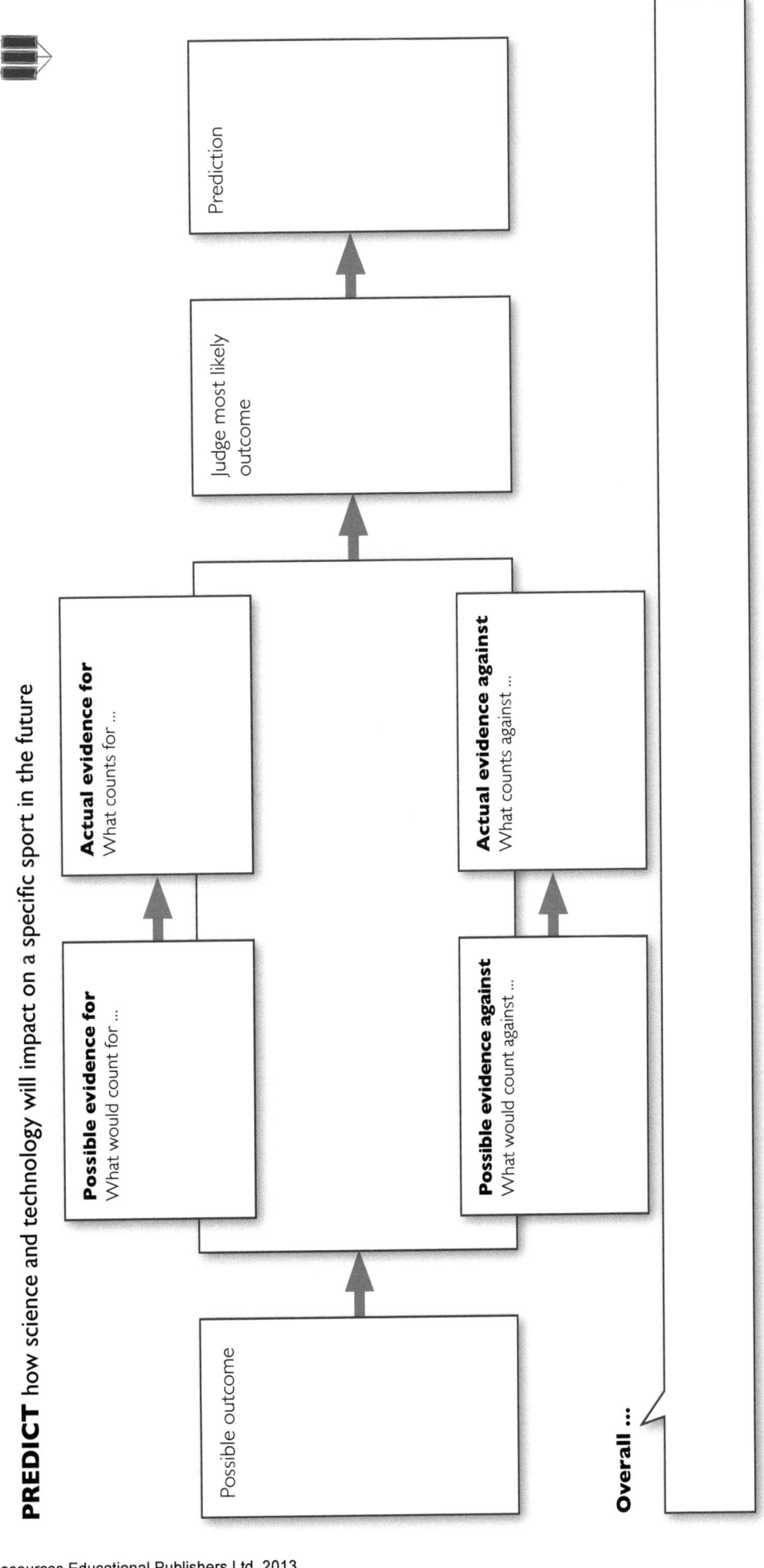

Overall …

© HookED, Pam Hook, 2013. All rights reserved. Adapted from HOT SOLO Predict map with permission ©Hooked on Thinking, 2004.

Table 1.3: HOT SOLO Predict rubric – future impact of science technology on sport

SOLO level	Success criteria		Student exemplar
	Visual map	**Text**	
Extended abstract		… and I make a generalisation judging the strength of the prediction.	… Overall I think that it's extremely likely that iPads will improve swimming performance. I found this article that supports my ideas about iPads improving performance in swimming: www.zdnet.com/what-olympic-sports-use-the-most-mobile-technology-7000001746
Relational		… and I give reasons or explain why this evidence supports or negates the predicted outcome …	… This means that swimmers and coaches can fine-tune performance instantly instead of waiting for access to video footage and it is accessible to more than just the elite athletes. …
Multistructural		… and I give evidence (possible and actual) in support of the outcome and evidence (possible and actual) that might negate the predicted outcome …	… In addition, there are plenty of apps (eg, Coach's Eye) to enhance coaching, and it is cost effective. … They may also hinder the "natural" ability of the athlete. …
Unistructural		My prediction identifies a possible outcome and supports it with evidence (possible and actual) in support of the predicted outcome …	iPads will improve swimming performance because you can analyse performance instantly on the poolside. … They may have a negative impact if the analysis used is poor. …
Prestructural		I need help to test a possible outcome.	I predict that iPads will improve swimming performance but I'm not sure how.

My learning outcome is _____ because _____
My next step is to _____

© HookED, Pam Hook, 2013. All rights reserved.
Adapted from HOT Predict self assessment rubric with permission ©Hooked on Thinking, 2004.

Learning focus: Sequence the stages of learning a new skill

Figure 1.3: HOT SOLO Sequence map – stages of skill learning

SEQUENCE the stages of learning a new skill

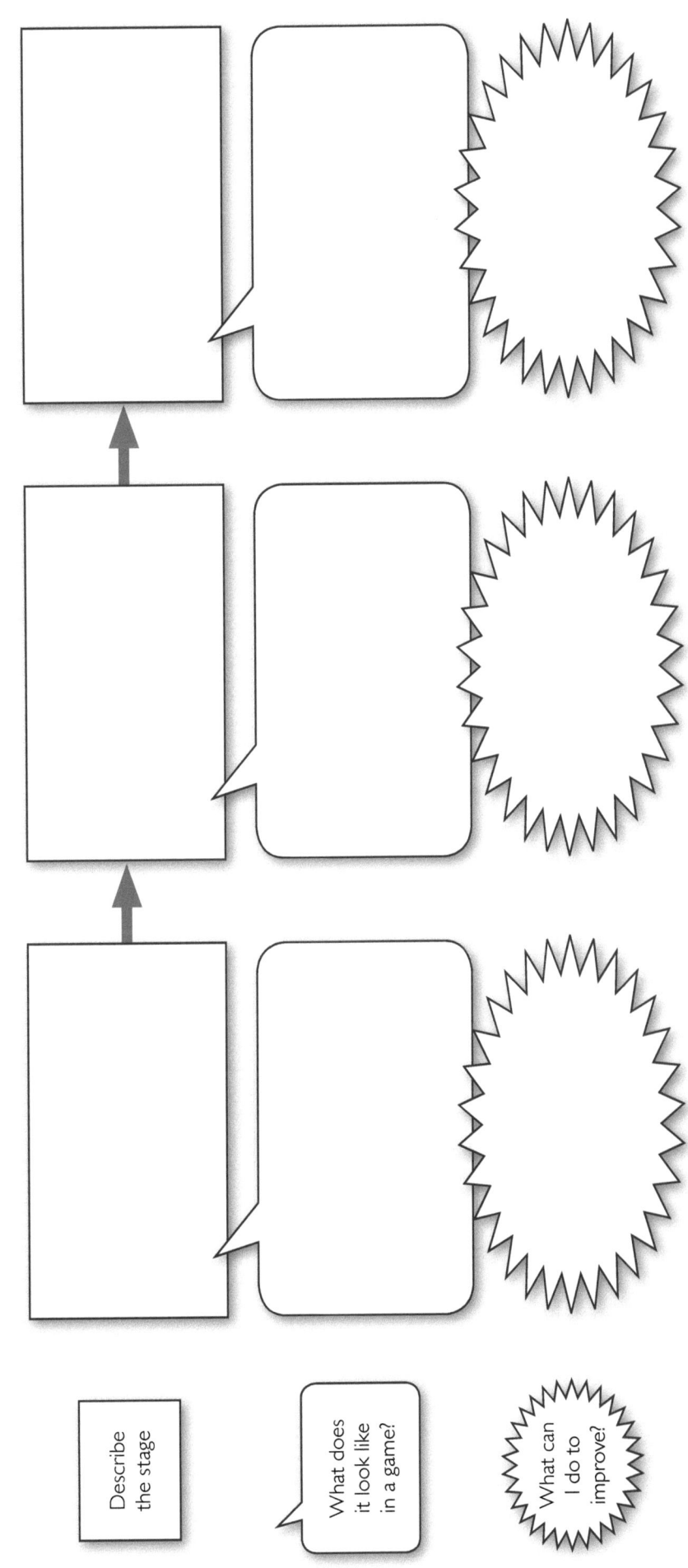

Table 1.4: HOT SOLO Sequence rubric – stages of skill learning

SOLO level	Success criteria		Student exemplar
	Visual map	**Text**	
Extended abstract		My statement identifies the idea to be sequenced, the relevant stages and the order of the stages; and explains the order of the stages; and includes a generalisation or prediction about the sequence.	… To help a beginner you need to give them lots of practice and demonstrations and keep the feedback very simple.
Relational		My statement identifies the idea to be sequenced, the relevant stages and the order of the stages; and explains the order of the stages.	… In the first stage a person is learning the new skill and makes lots of mistakes. Their brain is filled up with learning the technique of the skill. [+ explains later stages] …
Multistructural		My statement identifies the idea to be sequenced, the relevant stages and the order of the stages.	There are three stages of learning a new skill – beginner (cognitive), intermediate (associative) and advanced (autonomous). …
Unistructural		My statement identifies the idea to be sequenced and several stages or steps.	The first stage of learning is beginner (cognitive).
Prestructural		I need help to sequence.	Are there stages of learning a new skill? Don't you just learn it?

My learning outcome is _____ because _____
My next step is to _____

© HookED, Pam Hook, 2013. All rights reserved.
Adapted from HOT SOLO Sequence self assessment rubric with permission ©Hooked on Thinking, 2004.

Learning focus: Explain the cause and effect of errors in a skill

Figure 1.4: **HOT SOLO Explain Cause and Effect map – explain errors**

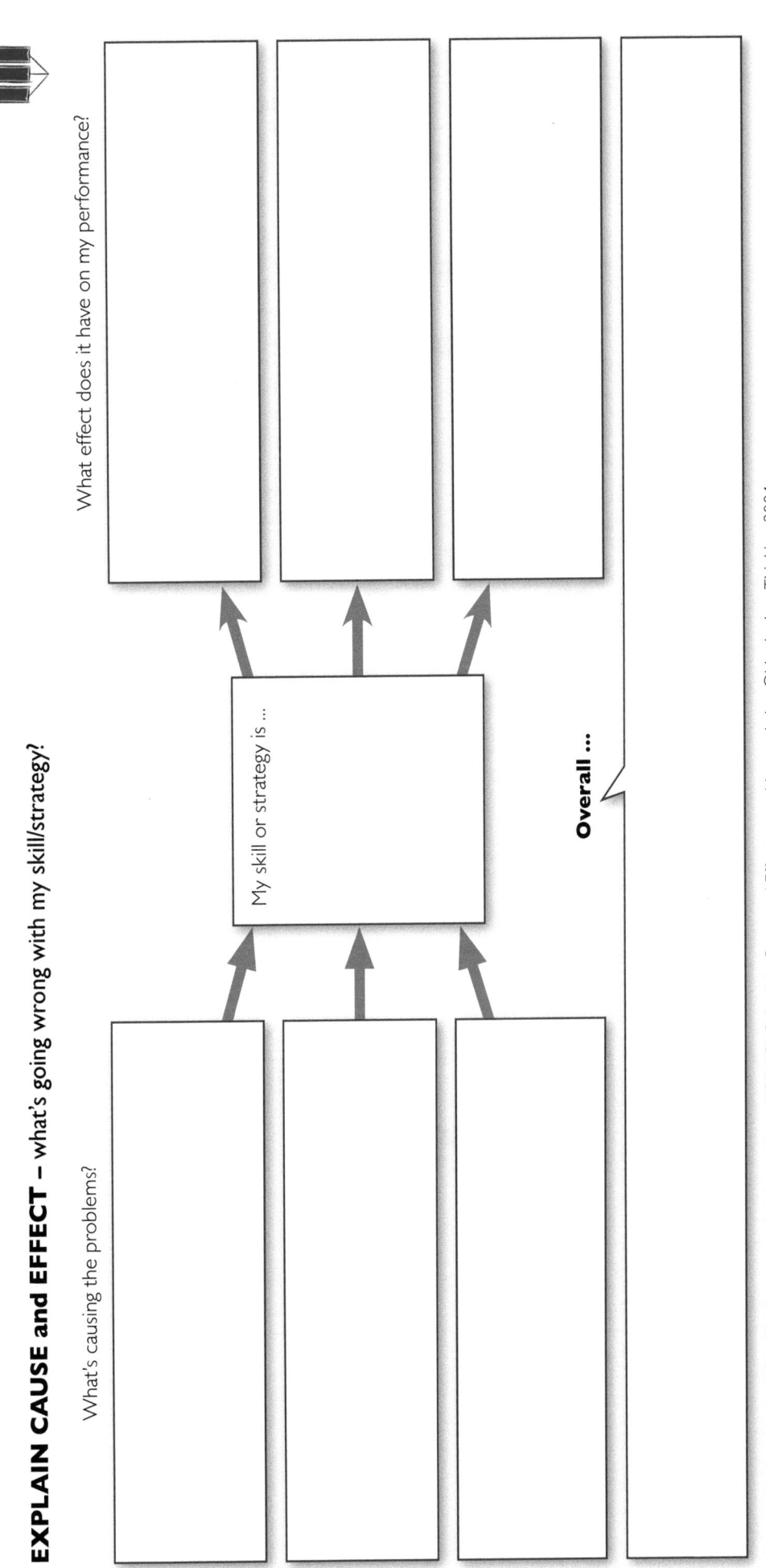

Table 1.5: HOT SOLO Explain Cause and Effect rubric – explain errors

SOLO level	Success criteria – Visual map	Success criteria – Text	Student exemplar
Extended abstract	[visual map with "Because" arrows feeding into a central box and out to effects, with summary bar "Overall I think... because... because..."]	My causal explanation identifies the event and several relevant causes or effects; and explains or gives reasons why something is a cause or an effect; and looks at the event in a new way.	… If I took more time before I shot (perhaps counting to 3) and made sure my feet were at least a shoulder width apart, I think I would be more consistent.
Relational	[visual map with "Because" arrows feeding into a central box and out to effects]	My causal explanation identifies the event and several relevant causes or effects; and explains or gives reasons why something is a cause or an effect.	My netball shots miss because I am unbalanced; this is because my feet are too close together. …
Multistructural	[visual map with multiple causes/effects boxes around a central box]	My causal explanation identifies the event and several relevant causes or effects.	… I also rush when I shoot. …
Unistructural	[visual map with one cause and one effect around a central box]	My causal explanation identifies the event and a relevant cause or effect.	My netball shots always miss because I am unbalanced when I release the ball. …
Prestructural	[empty visual map]	I need help to make a causal explanation.	I don't know what is wrong with my netball shot.

My learning outcome is _____ because _____

My next step is to _____

© HookED, Pam Hook, 2013. All rights reserved.
Adapted from HOT SOLO Explain Cause and Effect self assessment rubric with permission ©Hooked on Thinking, 2004.

Using SOLO functioning knowledge rubrics

The following SOLO functioning knowledge rubrics encourage students to reflect on their own progress and to be proactive when looking for strategies and approaches to advise their next steps.

The first SOLO functioning knowledge rubric (Table 1.6) provides an overview or generic template that can be used in many different movement contexts. There is space at the end of each row where you can add further attributes if you choose. Examples of more specific functioning knowledge rubrics follow (Tables 1.7–1.12).

Table 1.6: SOLO functioning knowledge rubric for movement skills – fundamental movement skills and strategy

Movement skills	Examples of student progress	Next steps
Unistructural	Unable to perform skills in closed environment. Struggles to participate in open drills and minor games. Makes many errors. Is inconsistent in focus	
Multistructural	Can perform skills in closed drills. Unable to use "right" skill in right situation in open drill / minor game. Makes few errors in closed drills. Is generally focused.	
Relational	Can perform skills in open drills and minor games. Uses skills appropriately. Skills allow minor games to flow successfully. Attempts to integrate strategy with skills. Makes few errors in open drill and minor games. Can identify errors but struggles to correct independently.	
Extended abstract	Can perform skills in games. Skills allow others to be involved in games. Uses skills with strategy successfully. Acts on feedback from external sources. Is beginning to identify own errors and corrects them.	

Table 1.7: SOLO functioning knowledge rubric for passing, throwing, force summation

Skill: Passing, throwing, force summation	Related skills: Body position; target identification; accuracy	Effective strategies, including strategies from students
Prestructural	I need help to pass effectively.	Show examples. Demonstrate. Give opportunities to practise.
Unistructural	I can pass a ball.	Give clear instructions (step by step). Prompt. Do situational teaching.
Multistructural	I can pass a ball in a closed environment (drill).	Revisit, recap, remind.
Relational	I can pass a ball in an open environment (moving drill or game).	Give repeated opportunities to practise.
Extended abstract	I can "read the game" and use a pass that is appropriate for the situation (look beyond me) consistently. I reflect on and refine my pass.	

Table 1.8: SOLO functioning knowledge rubric for receiving a pass

Skill: Receiving	Related skills: Body position; sighting the object; spatial awareness; stopping the object	Effective strategies, including strategies from students
Prestructural	I need help to receive the ball.	Show examples. Demonstrate. Give opportunities to practise.
Unistructural	I can receive a ball.	Give clear instructions (step by step). Prompt. Do situational teaching.
Multistructural	I can receive a ball in a closed environment (drill).	Revisit, recap, remind.
Relational	I can receive the ball in an open environment (moving drill or game).	Give repeated opportunities to practise.
Extended abstract	I can consistently "read the game" and move into space to receive a pass appropriately. I reflect on and refine my skill.	

Table 1.9: SOLO functioning knowledge rubric for moving well in different contexts

Skill: Moving in different contexts	Related skills: Spatial awareness; coordination; timing; motor skill (jumping, skipping …)	Effective strategies, including strategies from students
Prestructural	I need help to move well in different contexts.	Show examples. Demonstrate. Give opportunities to practise.
Unistructural	I can do basic movements in the way that the teacher demonstrates.	Give clear instructions (step by step). Prompt. Do situational teaching.
Multistructural	I can put together a simple sequence of movements (eg, long jump).	Revisit, recap, remind.
Relational	I can sequence specific movements together with success.	Give repeated opportunities to practise.
Extended abstract	I can put together an effective movement sequence, and reflect on and refine my performance.	

Table 1.10: SOLO functioning knowledge rubric for game sense – rules and fair play

Skill: Game sense – rules and fair play		Effective strategies, including strategies from students
Prestructural	I need help to learn and follow the rules of the game.	Show examples. Demonstrate. Give opportunities to practise.
Unistructural	I know the basic rules of the game.	Give clear instructions (step by step). Prompt. Do situational teaching.
Multistructural	I know the rules and I can apply them in a game.	Revisit, recap, remind.
Relational	I know the rules, I can apply them in a game and I can use them to play the game positively and fairly.	Give repeated opportunities to practise.
Extended abstract	I know the rules, I can apply them in a game and I can use them to play the game positively and fairly. I can refine my play and that of others, based on the rules.	

Table 1.11: SOLO functioning knowledge rubric for game sense – strategy

Skill: Game sense – strategy	**Related skills:** Attack; defence	**Effective strategies**, including strategies from students
Prestructural	I need help to play defence or attack.	Show examples. Demonstrate. Give opportunities to practise.
Unistructural	I can use attack or defensive strategy in a closed environment (drill).	Give clear instructions (step by step). Prompt. Do situational teaching.
Multistructural	I can use attack or defensive strategy in an open environment (modified game).	Revisit, recap, remind.
Relational	In a game situation I can use attack and defensive strategy at the right time and I understand the importance of this.	Give repeated opportunities to practise.
Extended abstract	In a game situation I can use attack and defensive strategy at the right time, I understand the importance of this and can reflect on and refine my own performance and that of others.	

Table 1.12: SOLO functioning knowledge rubric for game sense – positioning

Skill: Game sense – positioning		**Effective strategies**, including strategies from students
Prestructural	I need help to be in the right position during a game.	Show examples. Demonstrate. Give opportunities to practise.
Unistructural	I know the basic positions involved in the game.	Give clear instructions (step by step). Prompt. Do situational teaching.
Multistructural	I know the positions and can play in position in a game.	Revisit, recap, remind.
Relational	I know the positions and can play in position in a game, and I understand the importance of my position/role in the game.	Give repeated opportunities to practise.
Extended abstract	I know the positions and can play in position in a game. I understand the importance of my position/role in the game and can reflect on and refine the positional play of myself and others.	

Using SOLO stations

The following two examples of SOLO stations focus on gymnastics (Table 1.13) and netball (Table 1.14). Students work at their own pace through a series of SOLO-differentiated movement activities located in stations around the gymnasium or netball court. Self assessment and peer assessment rubrics at each station help determine when students are ready to move on.

Before the lesson starts, students complete a pre-test that identifies students who need small-group teaching before they start.

Table 1.13: SOLO station activities for gymnastics

Prestructural and unistructural station	Multistructural station
Use the skill cards and the help of your teacher to learn each skill.	Practise all your skills separately until you can confidently perform them. Use the YouTube videos to help you improve
Relational station	**Extended abstract station**
Sequence your skills to make a floor routine. Think about showcasing your skills and how you will put them together.	 Keep refining your routine and create a marking schedule for the floor routines to evaluate your performance and the performance of other groups.

Table 1.14: SOLO station activities for netball

Prestructural and unistructural station	Multistructural station
Use the skill cards and the help of your teacher to learn and practise passing, catching, shooting and defending. For example: www.mynetball.co.nz/community-netball/coaching/year-7-10/toolkit/skills/passing-a-catching/ball-control-activities.html	Practise your skills in moving drills. For example: www.mynetball.co.nz/community-netball/coaching/year-7-10/toolkit/skills/passing-a-catching/order-ball.html
Relational station	**Extended abstract station**
Link your skills in a game situation – think about movement and passing and receiving in space.	Create, practise and evaluate at least three different strategies for getting the ball from the defensive end to the goal circle.

Note: These activities could be adapted to other ball sports.

Using a SOLO learning log

This example (Table 1.15) shows how PE students can use a SOLO-coded self assessment rubric linked to a learning log to track their developing skills in touch rugby. For each lesson they fill out a learning log with the focus skill/strategy, the level they reached at the end of the lesson and how they will move forward.

Table 1.15: SOLO learning log for touch rugby

Prestructural	Unistructural	Multistructural	Relational	Extended abstract
I need help to pass effectively.	I can pass a touch ball.	I can pass a touch ball while moving.	I can use a range of passes in a game and I am consistent in my passing.	I can "read the game" and use a pass appropriate to the situation. I reflect on and refine my pass.
I need help to receive the ball.	I can receive a touch ball.	I can receive a touch ball while moving.	I can receive the ball in a range of situations in a game and my receiving is consistent.	I can "read the game" and move into space to receive a pass successfully. I reflect on and refine my skill.
I need help to play defence or attack.	I can tell you one attack or defensive strategy but I'm not sure when or where to use it.	I can use attack or defensive strategies in a game but I'm not sure why I use them.	In a game I can use attack and defensive strategies at the right time and I understand their importance …	… and I can reflect on and refine the performance of myself and others.
I need help to be in the right position during a game.	I know the basic positions (centre, link, wing) involved in the game.	I know the positions and can play in position in a game …	… and I understand the importance of my position/role in the game …	… and I can reflect on and refine the positional play of myself and others.
I need help with overall game play.	I have some basic skills and knowledge but struggle to use them in a game of touch.	I have the skills and game sense to participate in a game of touch but I'm still not sure what to do, when and why.	I can confidently and consistently use my skills and game sense to participate successfully in a game of touch and I make links between skills, strategy and performance …	… and I can reflect on and refine the skills and strategy of myself and others. I can create new plays. I am a role model for others.

My learning log reflection for touch   Date: _____

Today we worked on passing / receiving / attack/defence / positioning / overall game play (circle one).

I think I am at the _____ SOLO level for this aspect of touch because _____

_____

To move to the next level I need to _____

Teacher comment/assessment:

2. SOLO strategies for relationships with other people

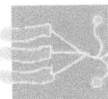

I like using SOLO maps in a group – we can share our ideas and come up with great questions.

Year 10 PE student

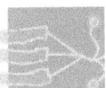

In [the relationships with other people strand,] students develop understandings, skills, and attitudes that enhance their interactions and relationships with others. (Ministry of Education 2007)

The relationships with other people strand is one of the unique aspects of the PE curriculum, providing opportunities for students to develop, practise, evaluate and understand interpersonal skills in "real life" situations in ways that are difficult to do in other learning areas. Students develop physical and social skills in relationships with others while they engage in physical play, games, sports and exercise in gyms and pools and on grass and turf; and in adventure and outdoor education activities such as tramping, camping, white-water rafting and mountaineering.

The learning intentions in Table 2.1 were developed through constructive alignment as examples of how this strand can be explored at a deep level. It is followed by two examples of effective SOLO strategies – SOLO maps and self assessment rubrics, and SOLO functioning knowledge rubrics – that can be used to encourage deeper thinking about and a deeper understanding of relationships with other people.

Effective SOLO strategies for relationships with other people

SOLO map

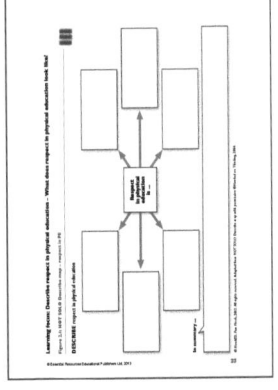

SOLO self assessment rubric

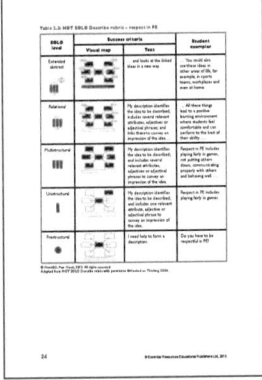

SOLO functioning knowledge rubric

Table 2.1: Possible learning intentions for exploring deep understanding of relationships with other people

Developed using constructive alignment

Unistructural and multistructural	Relational	Extended abstract
Identify the different roles in a team/group. *Identify* behaviours that enhance or detract from good group functioning. *Define* group. *Define* team. *Define* role. *Define* interpersonal skills. *Define* behaviour. *Define* participation. *Define* effective. *Define* assertiveness. *Describe* different roles in a team/group. *Describe* interpersonal skills. *Describe* respect in physical education. (See Figure 2.1, Table 2.2.) *List* successful teams/groups in our country. *List* effective behaviours. *List* detracting behaviours.	*Compare and contrast* successful groups with your own. (See Figure 2.3, Table 2.4.) *Analyse* (part–whole) key components of a successful team. *Apply* strategies for effective behaviour in groups/teams. *Classify* the roles and responsibilities in a team. *Explain the cause and effect* for a team that isn't functioning well. *Explain the cause and effect* for an individual's behaviour in relation to a group. *Describe+* discrimination. *Describe+* assertiveness in team activities. *Describe+* responsibility. *Describe+* features of an effective team. (See Figure 2.2, Table 2.3.)	*Evaluate* your use of strategies. *Evaluate* your group's performance in a task. *Evaluate* the success of your team. (See Figure 2.5, Table 2.6.) *Create* a set of "perfect" strategies for teams/groups. *Predict* how a team will perform based on its members' behaviour and interpersonal skills. *Describe++* strategies you use to be an effective team member. (See Figure 2.4, Table 2.5.) *Describe++* strategies for participation in a team or group.

Using SOLO maps and rubrics

The examples that follow show how SOLO maps and self assessment rubrics can be used to:

- describe what respect in PE looks like (Figure 2.1 and Table 2.2)
- describe and explain (Describe+) the features of an effective team (Figure 2.2 and Table 2.3)
- compare and contrast one's own team with an elite team (Figure 2.3 and Table 2.4)
- describe, explain and evaluate (Describe++) the strategies used to be an effective team member (Figure 2.4 and Table 2.5)
- evaluate the success of one's team (Figure 2.5 and Table 2.6).

Learning focus: Describe respect in physical education – What does respect in physical education look like?

Figure 2.1: HOT SOLO Describe map – respect in PE

DESCRIBE respect in physical education

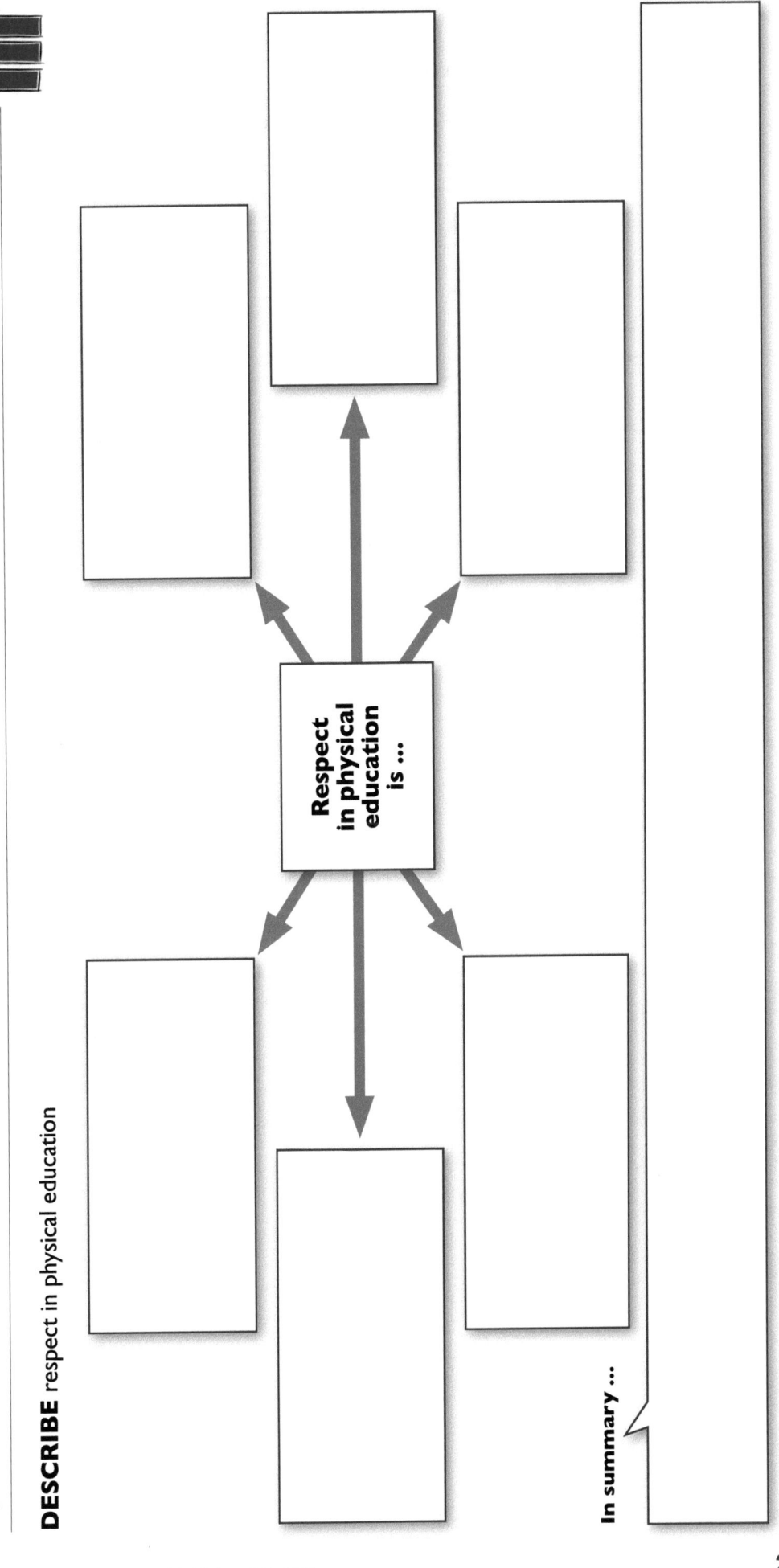

In summary …

© HookED, Pam Hook, 2013. All rights reserved. Adapted from HOT SOLO Describe map with permission ©Hooked on Thinking, 2004.

Table 2.2: HOT SOLO Describe rubric – respect in PE

SOLO level	Success criteria — Visual map	Success criteria — Text	Student exemplar
Extended abstract		… and looks at the linked ideas in a new way.	… You could also use these ideas in other areas of life, for example, in sports teams, workplaces and even at home.
Relational		My description identifies the idea to be described; includes several relevant attributes, adjectives or adjectival phrases; and links these to convey an impression of the idea …	… All these things lead to a positive learning environment where students feel comfortable and can perform to the best of their ability. …
Multistructural		My description identifies the idea to be described; and includes several relevant attributes, adjectives or adjectival phrases to convey an impression of the idea.	Respect in PE includes playing fairly in games, not putting others down, communicating properly with others and behaving well. …
Unistructural		My description identifies the idea to be described; and includes one relevant attribute, adjective or adjectival phrase to convey an impression of the idea.	Respect in PE includes playing fairly in games.
Prestructural		I need help to form a description.	Do you have to be respectful in PE?

© HookED, Pam Hook, 2013. All rights reserved.
Adapted from HOT SOLO Describe rubric with permission ©Hooked on Thinking, 2004.

Learning focus: Describe and explain (Describe+) the features of an effective team or group

Figure 2.2: HookED SOLO Describe+ map – describe and explain features of an effective team

DESCRIBE+ features of an effective team

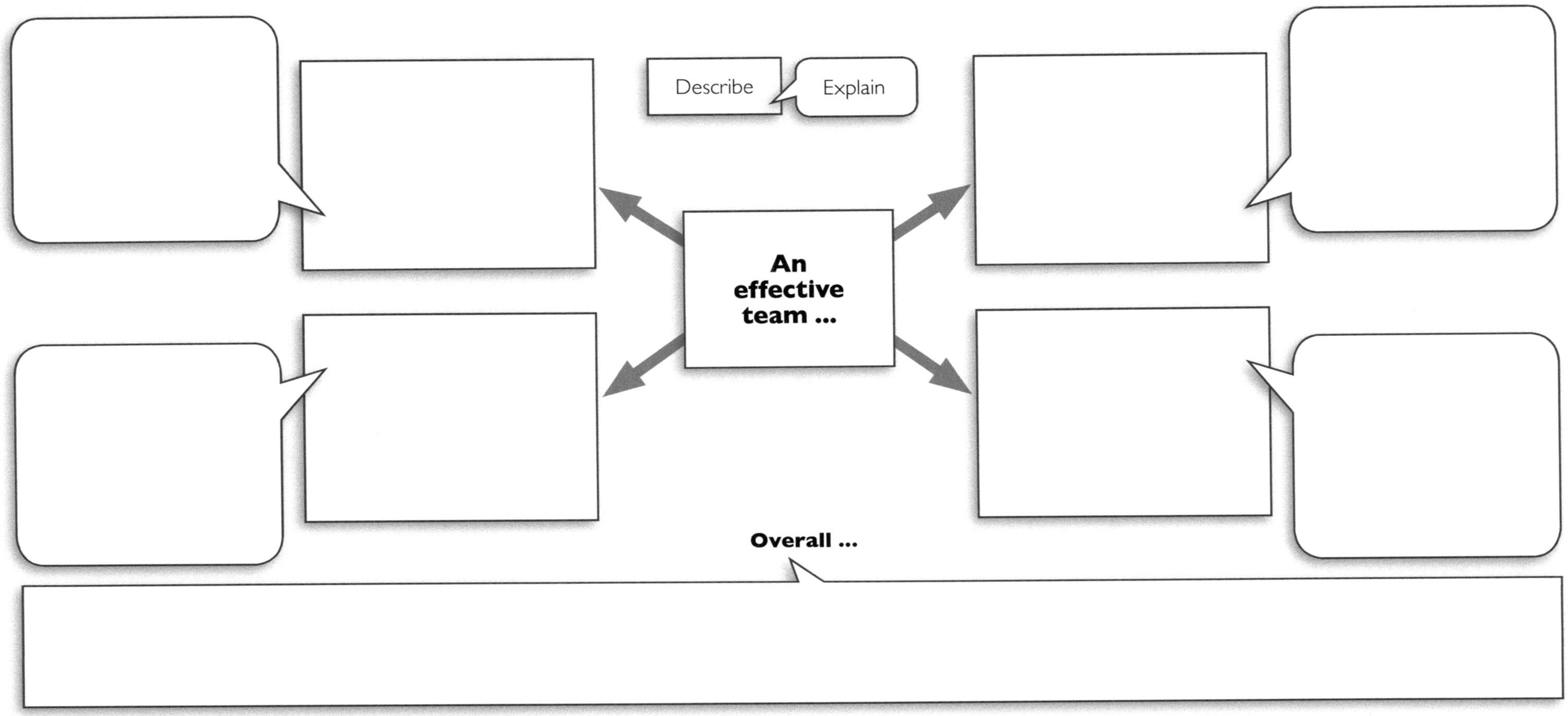

An effective team …

Describe | Explain

Overall …

Table 2.3: HookED SOLO Describe+ map – describe and explain features of an effective team

SOLO level	Success criteria – Visual map	Success criteria – Text	Student exemplar
Extended abstract		… and makes a generalisation that looks at the idea in a new way.	… Overall, building a great team is similar to building a great country. This is because the process is all about creating a sense of belonging to something with bigger goals.
Relational		My description identifies the idea to be described; includes several relevant attributes, adjectives or adjectival phrases; and explains why these are relevant to convey an impression of the idea …	… This is because these characteristics build a group culture or way of doing things where every member feels respected, listened to and valued, and every member gains something from belonging. …
Multistructural		My description identifies the idea to be described; and includes several relevant attributes, adjectives or adjectival phrases to convey an impression of the idea.	An effective team has clear goals, a collaborative culture, an openness to disagreements and an ability to resolve conflict. …
Unistructural		My description identifies the idea to be described; and includes one relevant attribute, adjective or adjectival phrase to convey an impression of the idea.	An effective team has clear goals.
Prestructural		I need help to form a description.	Does a team need to be effective?

© HookED, Pam Hook, 2013. All rights reserved.

Learning focus: Compare and contrast our team with an elite team – how is our team similar to and different from the Breakers (or All Blacks etc)?

Figure 2.3: HOT SOLO Compare and Contrast map – own team and elite sports team

COMPARE and CONTRAST our team with an elite sports team

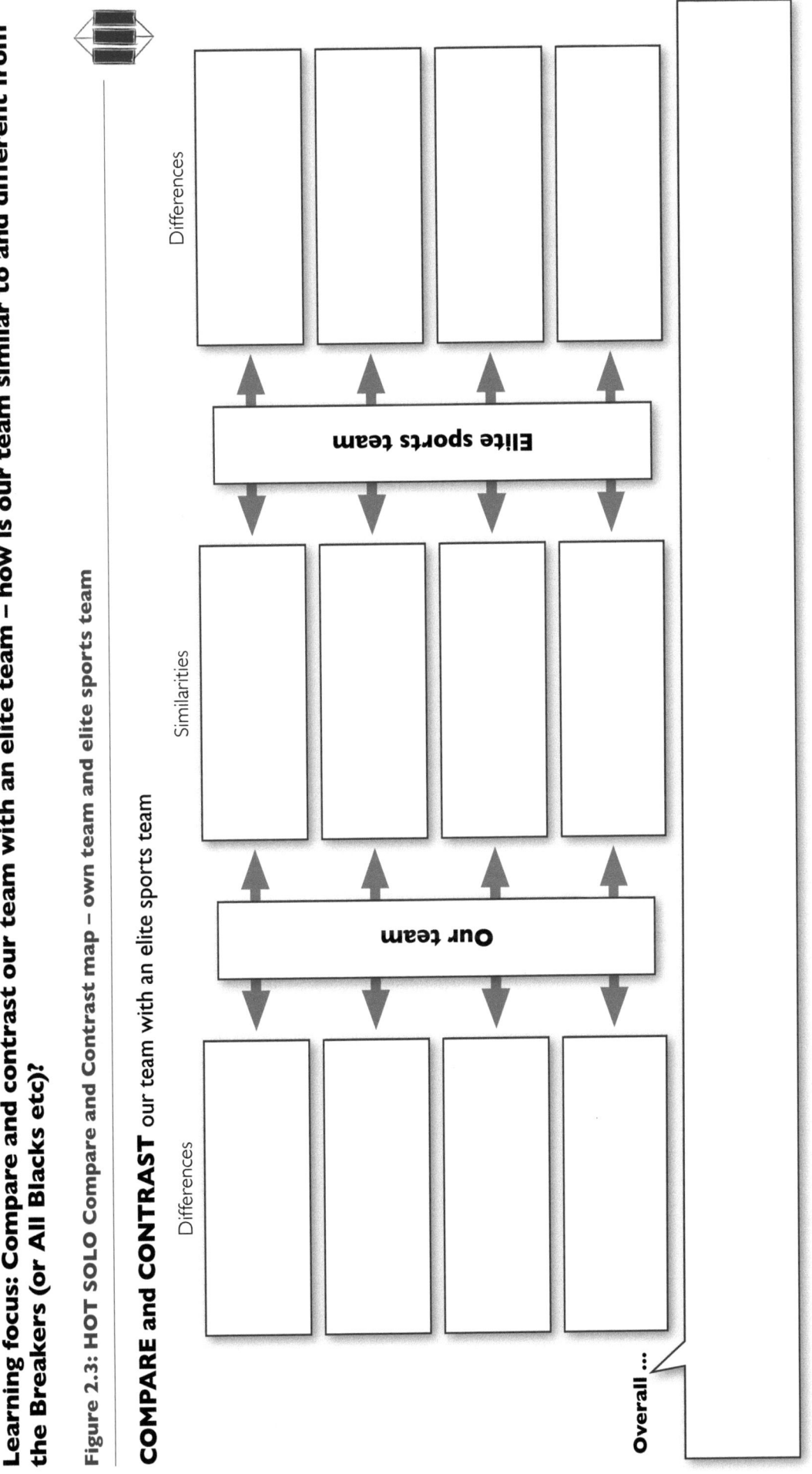

Table 2.4: HOT SOLO Compare and Contrast rubric – own team and elite sports team

SOLO level	Success criteria		Student exemplar
	Visual map	Text	
Extended abstract		… and makes a generalisation.	… Overall although we might seem very different I think our similarities are greater than our differences. This is because we both share the characteristics of what makes an effective team.
Relational		… and explains why they are relevant to the whole …	The Breakers team is similar to our team in several ways: we both have a clear purpose, set demanding performance goals and have discussion where everyone is heard. This is because we are both effective teams and have established a culture of working together for the good of the group. We are different in the amount of time we have for training and the number of people who turn out to watch the games. This is because the Breakers are a professional basketball team and have a huge following while we are the school B team. …
Multistructural		My comparison identifies several relevant similarities or differences …	The Breakers team is similar to our team in several ways: we both have a clear purpose, set demanding performance goals and have discussion where everyone is heard. We are different in the amount of time we have for training and the number of people who turn out to watch the games.
Unistructural		My comparison identifies one relevant similarity or difference.	The Breakers team is similar to our team in that we both have a clear purpose.
Prestructural		I need help to form a comparison.	

© HookED, Pam Hook, 2013. All rights reserved. Adapted from HOT SOLO Compare and Contrast self assessment rubric with permission ©Hooked on Thinking, 2004.

Learning focus: Describe, explain and evaluate (Describe++) the strategies you use to be an effective team member

Figure 2.4: HookED SOLO Describe++ map – describe, explain and evaluate strategies for being an effective team member

DESCRIBE++ the strategies you use to be an effective team member

Strategies

Describe the strategy

Explain why it's effective

Where else could you use it

Overall …

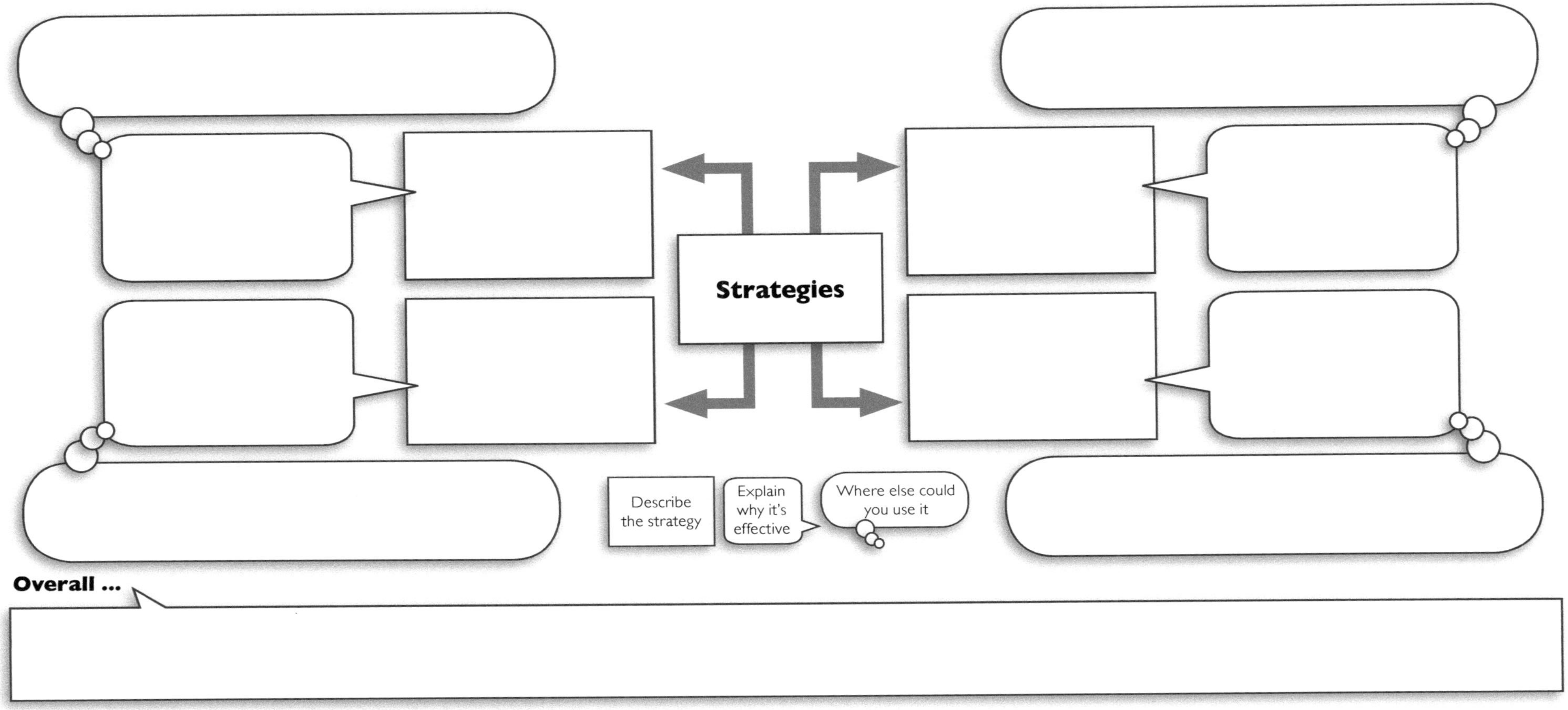

© HookED, Pam Hook, 2013. All rights reserved.

Table 2.5: HookED SOLO Describe++ rubric – describe, explain and evaluate strategies for being an effective team member

SOLO level	Success criteria		Student exemplar
	Visual map	**Text**	
Extended abstract		I can describe several relevant attributes, adjectives or adjectival phrases; explain these, giving reasons why; and evaluate them to convey an impression of the idea.	… Overall I think these strategies worked together to make me a highly effective team player because they all focused on what was best for the team, for example …
Relational		I can describe several relevant attributes, adjectives or adjectival phrases; and explain these, giving reasons why to convey an impression of the idea.	… I did these things because an effective team relies on the actions of all of its members. This is because in an effective team you have to be able to participate and contribute in ways that improve group outcomes rather than "what is best for me" outcomes. …
Multistructural		I can describe several relevant attributes, adjectives or adjectival phrases to convey an impression of the idea.	To be an effective team member I made sure I went to every training session even if I didn't need to learn the new skill; I showed up for every game even if I wasn't playing; and I worked with and supported others to get the best outcome for the team as a whole, even though this meant that sometimes I had to pass and let someone else score the winning goal. …
Unistructural		I can describe one relevant attribute, adjective or adjectival phrase to convey an impression of the idea.	To be an effective team member I made sure I went to every training session and showed up for every game.
Prestructural		I need help to describe, explain and evaluate.	I was in the team, if that is what you are asking.

© HookED, Pam Hook, 2013. All rights reserved.

Learning focus: Evaluate the success of your team – how successful was your team; to what extent was your team successful?

Figure 2.5: **HOT SOLO Evaluate map – team success**

EVALUATE the success of your team

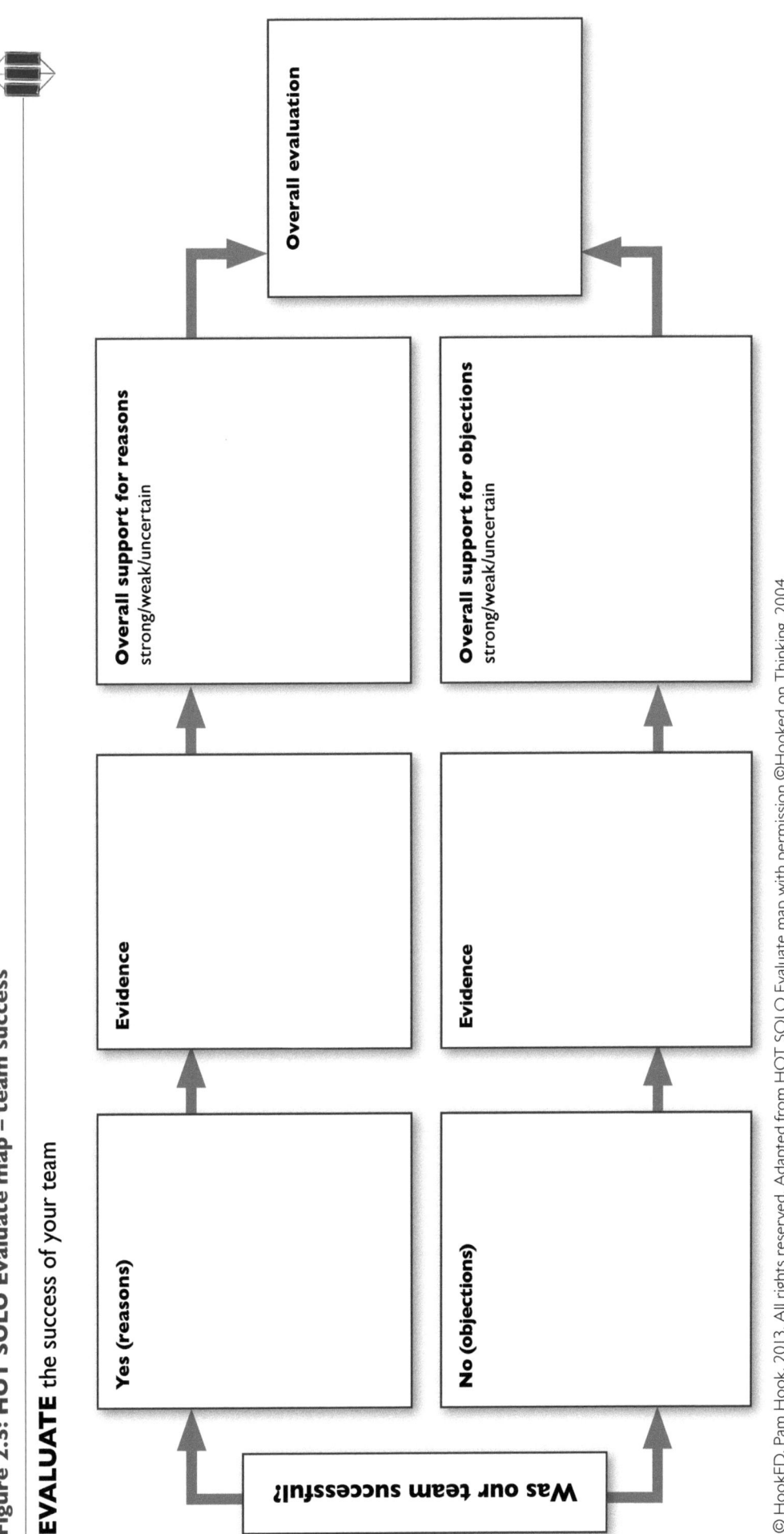

Table 2.6: HOT SOLO Evaluate rubric – team success

SOLO level	Success criteria		Student exemplar
	Visual map	**Text**	
Extended abstract		… and it checks the reliability and validity of facts in the reasons and objections. It judges the reasons and objections individually and collectively and forms a generalisation.	… Even though we had a good winning record, our team wasn't really successful as it wasn't inclusive and not everyone felt happy all of the time – which was the main objective of the lessons.
Relational		… and explains why these reasons support it; and explains why these objections work against it …	We won six out of the eight games in the tournament – a good success rate. At times the teacher had to remind us about subbing players and I heard three players in my team making negative comments about others. …
Multistructural		My evaluation identifies the argument; and gives reasons for *and* objections to the argument …	However, there were a lot of putdowns and some people were left on the side a lot. …
Unistructural		My evaluation identifies the argument; and gives reasons for *or* objections to the argument.	I think my team was successful because we won most of our games. …
Prestructural		I need help to make an evaluation.	I don't know whether my team was successful or not!

© HookED, Pam Hook, 2013. All rights reserved.

Using SOLO functioning knowledge rubrics

The following SOLO functioning knowledge rubrics encourage students to reflect on their own progress and to be proactive when looking for strategies and approaches to advise their next steps. Useful in health classes as well as PE, they cover functioning knowledge in the following areas:

- relationships (Tables 2.7–2.10)
- identity, sensitivity and respect (Tables 2.11–2.13)
- interpersonal skills (Tables 2.14–2.18).

Learning focus: Relationships

Table 2.7: SOLO functioning knowledge rubric for listening and responding

Relationships: Listen and respond	**Related skills:** Pause before responding, be trustworthy, take time, adapt your idea to fit with others' ideas, focus, pay attention to non-verbal cues, listen to understand, be open-minded, follow up, seek feedback	**Effective strategies**, including strategies from students
Prestructural	I need help to communicate with and/or listen to others. I lack a self-awareness of my impact on others.	Show examples. Demonstrate. Give opportunities to practise.
Unistructural	I can communicate with others if I am prompted or reminded. I can listen to others if I am prompted or reminded.	Give clear instructions (step by step). Prompt. Do situational teaching.
Multistructural	I can communicate ideas and relate to others. I can listen to the ideas of others and respond to them …	Revisit, recap, remind.
Relational	… and I can explain these ideas clearly and effectively. I can actively listen to others and respond appropriately, reflecting a personal understanding of the viewpoint expressed.	Give repeated opportunities to practise.
Extended abstract	I can balance listening and responding. I can synthesise what I hear and evaluate or elaborate on in response to others' ideas, offering alternative perspectives.	

Table 2.8: SOLO functioning knowledge rubric for relationships with individuals or groups

Relationships: Individuals or groups		**Effective strategies**, including strategies from students
Prestructural	I need help to work in a group (with teachers or other students)	Show examples. Demonstrate. Give opportunities to practise.
Unistructural	I can work in a group with my friends.	Give clear instructions (step by step). Prompt. Do situational teaching.
Multistructural	I can work in a group with anyone in my class, year level or team …	Revisit, recap, remind.
Relational	… and respond positively to the needs of others …	Give repeated opportunities to practise.
Extended abstract	… and reflect on how well I work with the group and seek feedback on how I can improve.	

Table 2.9: SOLO functioning knowledge rubric for teamwork

Relationships: Teamwork	**Related skills:** Take part, treat each member with respect, value all contributions, don't take comments personally, work together	**Effective strategies**, including strategies from students
Prestructural	I need help to interact with others. I need help to participate in a team.	Show examples. Demonstrate. Give opportunities to practise.
Unistructural	I can interact with others one-to-one. I can participate in a team.	Give clear instructions (step by step). Prompt. Do situational teaching.
Multistructural	I can interact with others in a small group. I can participate and take responsibility in a team.	Revisit, recap, remind.
Relational	I can interact with others in a team, adopting different roles to meet different demands. I can participate and take responsibility in a team and explain my choices in terms of team outcomes.	Give repeated opportunities to practise.
Extended abstract	I can interact confidently with others in a team, and make individual compromises based on identifying ways to improve team outcomes. I can participate in creating healthy teams by taking responsibility and critical action.	

Table 2.10: SOLO functioning knowledge rubric for positivity

Relationships: Positivity	**Related skills:** Work with others, showing joy, gratitude, serenity, interest, hope, pride, amusement, inspiration, awe and love	**Effective strategies**, including strategies from students
Prestructural	I need help to work with others in a positive way.	Show examples. Demonstrate. Give opportunities to practise.
Unistructural	I can work with a friend positively. I can work on a familiar task positively.	Give clear instructions (step by step). Prompt. Do situational teaching.
Multistructural	I can work with people I know positively. I can work on different tasks – familiar and unfamiliar – positively.	Revisit, recap, remind.
Relational	I can work with people I know and people I don't know positively. I can adjust my behaviour and take different roles to help the group work together.	Give repeated opportunities to practise.
Extended abstract	I can work with anyone positively. To help the group work together more positively, I can: • adjust my behaviour and roles • evaluate how the group is working and suggest different roles.	

Learning focus: Identity, sensitivity and respect

Table 2.11: SOLO functioning knowledge rubric for showing respect

Identity, sensitivity and respect: Showing respect	**Related skills:** Show respect through greetings, manners, kindness, and appropriate eye contact	**Effective strategies**, including strategies from students
Prestructural	I need help to know what showing respect is like.	Show examples. Demonstrate. Give opportunities to practise.
Unistructural	I know what showing respect is and can show respect when I am reminded to.	Give clear instructions (step by step). Prompt. Do situational teaching.
Multistructural	I know what showing respect is and can show respect when I am with others …	Revisit, recap, remind.
Relational	… and I can explain why I behave in a respectful way to others …	Give repeated opportunities to practise.
Extended abstract	… and I can help others to understand why showing respect is a good thing by the way I behave (role model).	

Table 2.12: SOLO functioning knowledge rubric for self awareness

Identity, sensitivity and respect: Self awareness	**Related skills:** Having a clear perception of your personality, strengths, weaknesses, thoughts, beliefs, motivation and emotions	**Effective strategies**, including strategies from students
Prestructural	I need someone to tell me how well I am doing when I am working with a team (evaluating).	Show examples. Demonstrate. Give opportunities to practise.
Unistructural	I can tell how well I am doing when I am working with a team if someone helps me.	Give clear instructions (step by step). Prompt. Do situational teaching.
Multistructural	I can tell how well I am doing when I am working with a team.	Revisit, recap, remind.
Relational	I can judge how well I am doing when I am working with a team, and change things to improve the teamwork.	Give repeated opportunities to practise.
Extended abstract	In response to changes in my team environment, I can: • plan, monitor and evaluate my progress intuitively • adjust my strategies.	

Table 2.13: SOLO functioning knowledge rubric for empathy

Identity, sensitivity and respect: Empathy	**Related skills:** Caring for others, wanting to help others, experiencing emotions that match others' emotions, sensing what the other person is thinking or feeling	**Effective strategies**, including strategies from students
Prestructural	I have an opinion.	Show examples. Demonstrate. Give opportunities to practise.
Unistructural	I understand that other people have different opinions to mine.	Give clear instructions (step by step). Prompt. Do situational teaching.
Multistructural	I understand that my opinion is one of many different viewpoints. I can identify other people's opinions.	Revisit, recap, remind.
Relational	I understand that my opinion is influenced by many different viewpoints. I can explain how these different viewpoints have influenced my opinion.	Give repeated opportunities to practise.
Extended abstract	I understand that my opinion is influenced by many different viewpoints. I can empathise with others' viewpoints and evaluate how they influence my opinion.	

Learning focus: Interpersonal skills

Table 2.14: SOLO functioning knowledge rubric for communication (listening and responding)

Interpersonal skills: Communication (listening and responding)	Related skills: Express your ideas clearly, listen carefully, make relevant comments or responses, and show you agree, disagree or neither agree or disagree	Effective strategies, including strategies from students
Prestructural	I can share my ideas with the group.	Show examples. Demonstrate. Give opportunities to practise.
Unistructural	I can share my ideas with the group and listen to the ideas of others.	Give clear instructions (step by step). Prompt. Do situational teaching.
Multistructural	I can share my ideas with the group, and listen to and respond to the ideas of others.	Revisit, recap, remind.
Relational	I can share my ideas with the group, and listen to and respond to the ideas of others by comparing my ideas with other ideas expressed by the group …	Give repeated opportunities to practise.
Extended abstract	… and I can evaluate the progress of group discussion and suggest new directions.	

Table 2.15: SOLO functioning knowledge rubric for conflict resolution

Interpersonal skills: Conflict resolution	Related skills: Be aware and respectful of differences, remain calm and alert, keep control over your emotions and behaviour, pay attention to the feelings being expressed	Effective strategies, including strategies from students
Prestructural	I need help to resolve a dispute.	Show examples. Demonstrate. Give opportunities to practise.
Unistructural	I ask for help to resolve a dispute.	Give clear instructions (step by step). Prompt. Do situational teaching.
Multistructural	I can resolve a dispute by talking to the people involved …	Revisit, recap, remind.
Relational	… and finding a common position that everyone can agree on …	Give repeated opportunities to practise.
Extended abstract	… and I can reflect on the steps taken to resolve a dispute and how they might be improved if this situation arises again.	

Table 2.16: SOLO functioning knowledge rubric for behaviour

Interpersonal skills: Behaviour	When addressing difficult behaviours: conflict, withdrawal, monopolising, blaming	Effective strategies, including strategies from students
Prestructural	I need help to know what you are talking about.	Show examples. Demonstrate. Give opportunities to practise.
Unistructural	I behave in a way that suits me, eg, I am who I am.	Give clear instructions (step by step). Prompt. Do situational teaching.
Multistructural	I behave in a way that suits me and I accept that they will act in a way that suits them, eg, I am who I am and they are who they are …	Revisit, recap, remind.
Relational	… However, if given clear guidelines I can adjust how I behave in response to who I am with …	Give repeated opportunities to practise.
Extended abstract	… and I seek feedback and review my behaviour when I am with others to see if I can be a better friend or group member.	

Table 2.17: SOLO functioning knowledge rubric for giving feedback

Interpersonal skills: Giving feedback	Related skills: Be timely, be specific, use "I" statements, limit the focus, include positives, provide specific suggestions, follow up, seek feedback	Effective strategies, including strategies from students
Prestructural	I need help to give feedback.	Show examples. Demonstrate. Give opportunities to practise.
Unistructural	I can give feedback.	Give clear instructions (step by step). Prompt. Do situational teaching.
Multistructural	I can give feedback and elaborate on it …	Revisit, recap, remind.
Relational	… and I can explain the impact or give reasons …	Give repeated opportunities to practise.
Extended abstract	… and I can suggest next steps and follow up. I can seek feedback on my feedback.	

Table 2.18: SOLO functioning knowledge rubric for assertiveness

Interpersonal skills: Assertiveness	Related skills: Respects the wants, needs and feelings of the other person; accepts that the other person may see things differently; works with the other person to find the answer; uses "I" statements, eg, "I feel ..." rather than "You never ..."; waits and listens to the other person; asks the other person to similarly give constructive feedback to the communicator in future; does not interrupt the other person	Effective strategies, including strategies from students
Prestructural	I need to [insert attribute of assertive behaviour].	Show examples. Demonstrate. Give opportunities to practise.
Unistructural	I ask for help to [insert attribute of assertive behaviour].	Give clear instructions (step by step). Prompt. Do situational teaching.
Multistructural	I can [insert attribute of assertive behaviour] in controlled environments (group activity, small group game).	Revisit, recap, remind.
Relational	I can [insert attribute of assertive behaviour] in a range of changing environments and with a range of people ...	Give repeated opportunities to practise.
Extended abstract	... and I can reflect on and refine my assertiveness when needed.	

3. SOLO strategies for healthy communities and environments

 I like how SOLO maps can make my thinking more organised.
Year 9 PE student

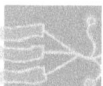 In [the healthy communities and environments strand,] students contribute to healthy communities and environments by taking responsible and critical action. (Ministry of Education 2007)

While many schools cover the healthy communities and environments strand of the curriculum in health, there are also opportunities in physical education to explore the social influences and issues related to physical activity. Contexts that can be used to explore this strand include Olympism and the impact of other major sporting events on society and participation in sport, investigating the local community facilities, fitness crazes, media and sport/physical activity and health promotion. These ideas play a major role in many senior physical education achievement standards and it is beneficial to encourage junior students to use SOLO as a model to start thinking more deeply in these contexts.

The learning intentions in Table 3.1 were developed through constructive alignment as examples of how this strand can be explored at a deep level. It is followed by a series of SOLO maps and self assessment rubrics that can be used to encourage deeper thinking about and a deeper understanding of healthy communities and environments.

Effective SOLO strategies for healthy communities and environments

SOLO maps

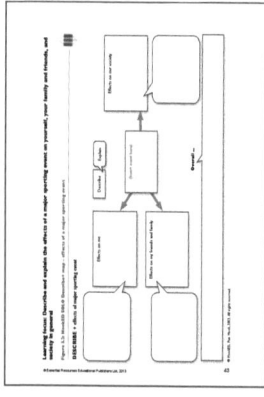

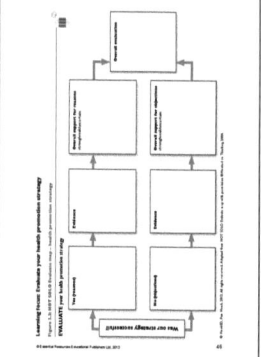

SOLO self assessment rubrics

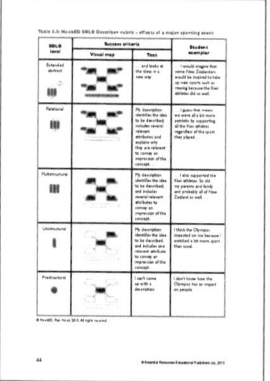

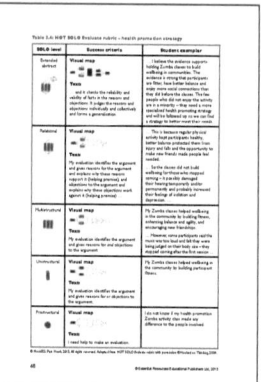

Table 3.1: Possible learning intentions for exploring deep understanding of healthy communities and environments

Developed using constructive alignment

Unistructural and multistructural 	Relational 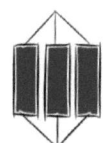	Extended abstract 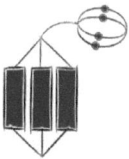
Identify barriers and enablers. *Define* lifestyle. *Define* wellbeing. *Define* society. *Define* sport. *Define* physical education. *Define* barriers and enablers. *Define* health promotion. *Describe* barriers and enablers. *Describe* a major sporting event. *Describe* different fitness crazes. *Describe* the impact of a major sporting event on sectors of society. *Describe* places to participate in physical activity in the community.	*Compare and contrast* different Olympic sports. *Compare and contrast* the impact of Olympics on different countries. *Compare and contrast* media coverage of different sports. *Compare and contrast* different community facilities. *Explain the cause and effect* of barriers to physical activity. (See Figure 3.1, Table 3.2.) *Explain the cause and effect* of enablers to physical activity. *Describe and explain* (Describe+) how media influence physical activity. *Describe and explain* (Describe+) the effects of a major sporting event on yourself, your family and friends, and society in general. (See Figure 3.2, Table 3.3.) *Describe and explain* (Describe+) health promotion strategies.	*Evaluate* the impact of the Olympics on society's wellbeing. *Predict* the long-term effect of a major sporting event on our society. *Create* a health promotion strategy. *Predict* the effects of your health promotion strategy. *Evaluate* your health promotion strategy. (See Figure 3.3, Table 3.4.) *Generalise* about the effects of a major sporting event on society's participation in physical activity. *Evaluate* a community facility.

Using SOLO maps

The examples that follow show how SOLO maps and self assessment rubrics can be used to:
- explain the cause and effect of barriers to participation in physical activity (Figure 3.1 and Table 3.2)
- describe and explain (Describe+) the effects of a major sporting event on yourself, your family and friends, and society in general (Figure 3.2 and Table 3.3)
- evaluate your health promotions strategy (Figure 3.3 and Table 3.4).

Learning focus: Explain the cause and effect of barriers to participation in physical activity

Figure 3.1: HOT SOLO Explain Cause and Effect map – barriers to participation in physical activity

EXPLAIN CAUSE and EFFECT – how do barriers affect participation?

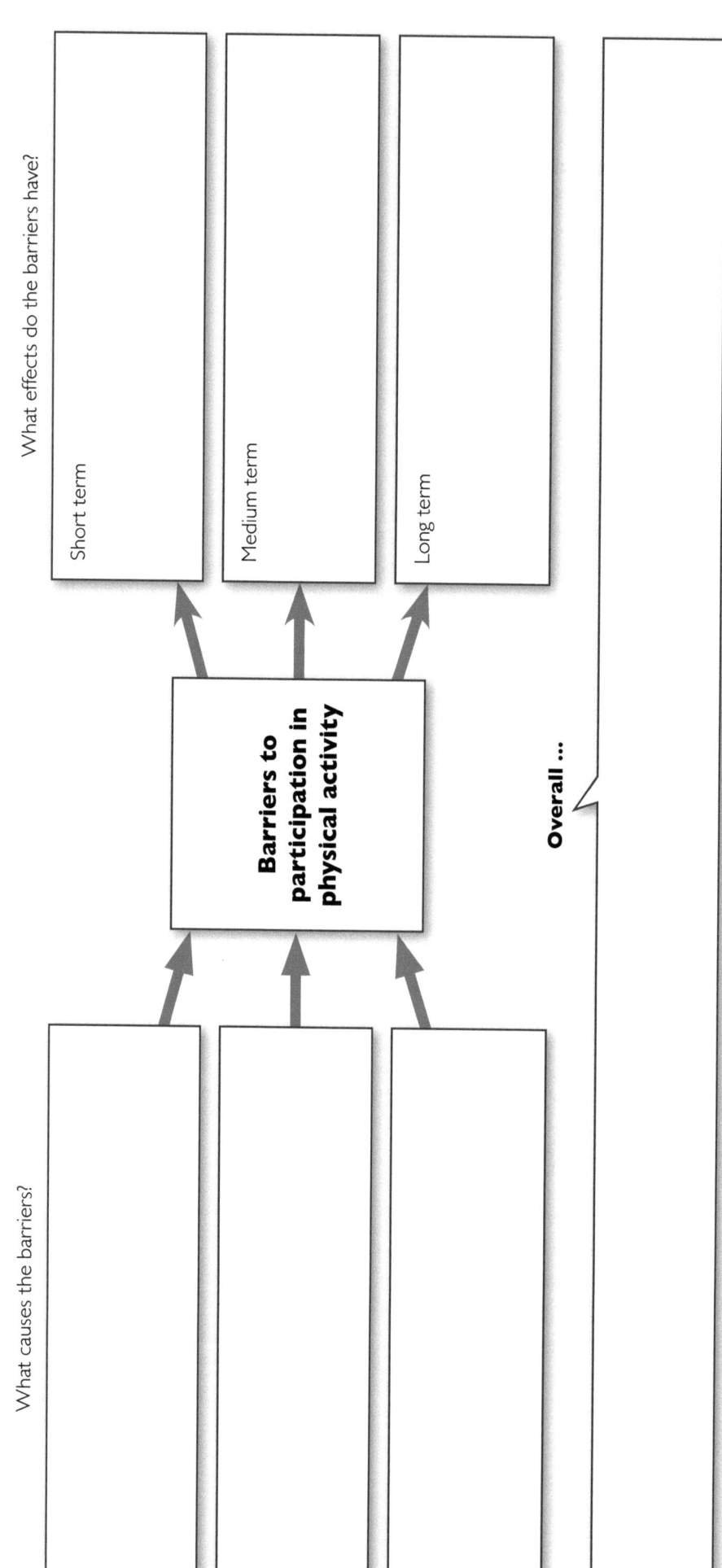

Table 3.2: HOT SOLO Explain Cause and Effect rubric – barriers to participation in physical activity

SOLO level	Success criteria – Visual map	Success criteria – Text	Student exemplar
Extended abstract	[Visual map with multiple "Because" nodes and "Overall I think... because... because..." summary]	… and looks at the event in a new way.	… Government could help to overcome some of these barriers by providing facilities for communities in need and helping athletes with fees and equipment.
Relational	[Visual map with multiple "Because" nodes connected]	… and explains or gives reasons why something is a cause or an effect …	The lack of facilities is a cause because it means there are fewer opportunities for physical activity. For example, in Christchurch after the earthquakes people have given up some sports because the facilities are gone (no athletics track, fewer swimming pools).
Multistructural	[Visual map with multiple nodes connected]	My causal explanation identifies the event and several relevant causes or effects …	Lack of facilities, lack of money and lack of family support could be barriers to physical activity. The effects would be that some people are unable to participate and the level of participation in physical activity may fall. …
Unistructural	[Visual map with one filled node connected]	My causal explanation identifies the event and a relevant cause or effect.	Lack of facilities is a barrier to physical activity because it means people are unable to participate in certain activities.
Prestructural	[Visual map with empty nodes]	I need help to make a causal explanation.	I know there are barriers to physical activity but I can't name one.

© HookED, Pam Hook, 2013. All rights reserved.
Adapted from HOT SOLO Explain Cause and Effect rubric with permission ©Hooked on Thinking, 2004.

Learning focus: Describe and explain the effects of a major sporting event on yourself, your family and friends, and society in general

Figure 3.2: HookED SOLO Describe+ map – effects of a major sporting event

DESCRIBE+ effects of major sporting event

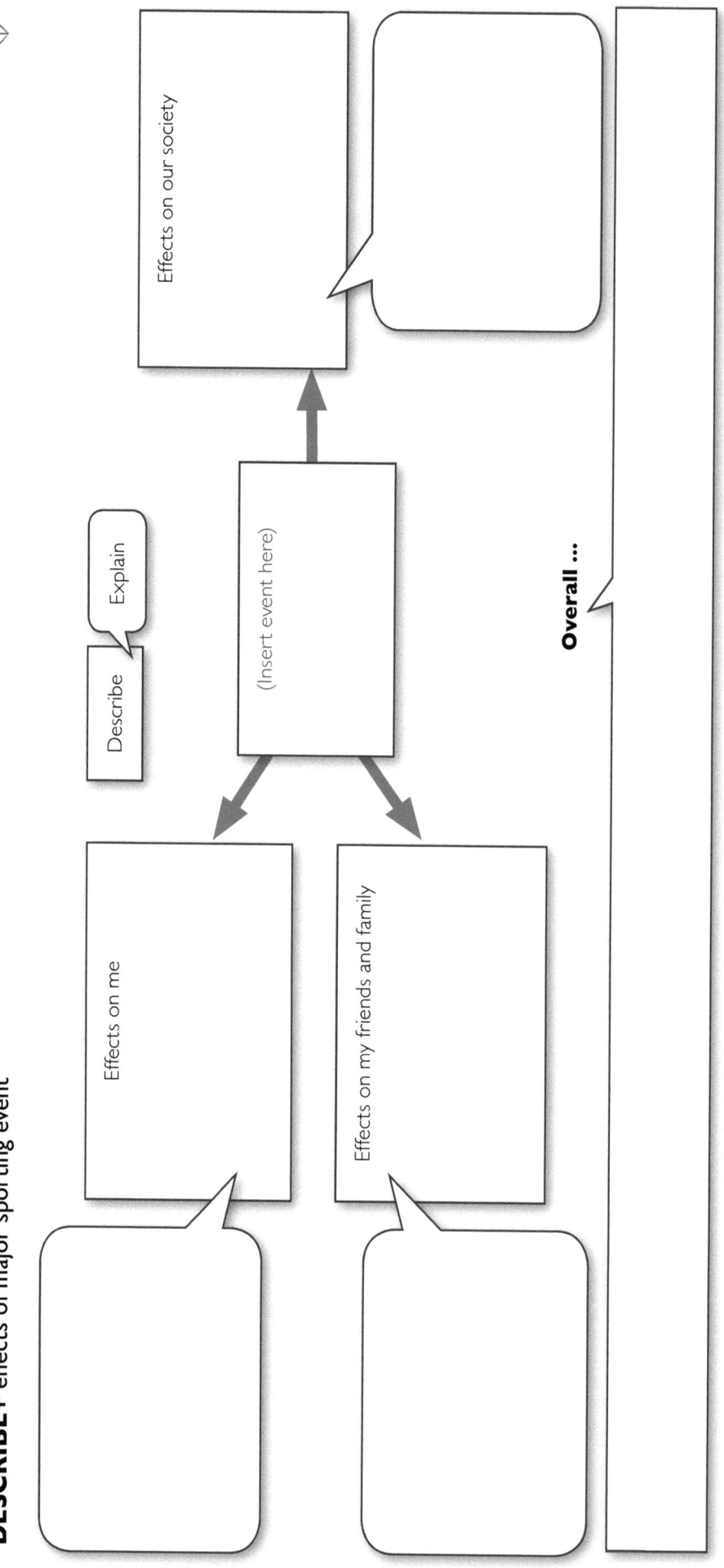

Table 3.3: HookED SOLO Describe+ rubric – effects of a major sporting event

SOLO level	Success criteria – Visual map	Success criteria – Text	Student exemplar
Extended abstract		… and looks at the ideas in a new way.	… I would imagine that some New Zealanders would be inspired to take up new sports such as rowing because the Kiwi athletes did so well.
Relational		My description identifies the idea to be described; includes several relevant attributes; and explains why they are relevant to convey an impression of the concept. …	… I guess that means we were all a bit more patriotic by supporting all the Kiwi athletes regardless of the sport they played. …
Multistructural		My description identifies the idea to be described; and includes several relevant attributes to convey an impression of the concept.	… I also supported the Kiwi athletes. So did my parents and family and probably all of New Zealand as well. …
Unistructural		My description identifies the idea to be described; and includes one relevant attribute to convey an impression of the concept.	I think the Olympics impacted on me because I watched a lot more sport than usual. …
Prestructural		I can't come up with a description.	I don't know how the Olympics has an impact on people.

© HookED, Pam Hook, 2013. All rights reserved.

Learning focus: Evaluate your health promotion strategy

Figure 3.3: HOT SOLO Evaluate map – health promotion strategy

EVALUATE your health promotion strategy

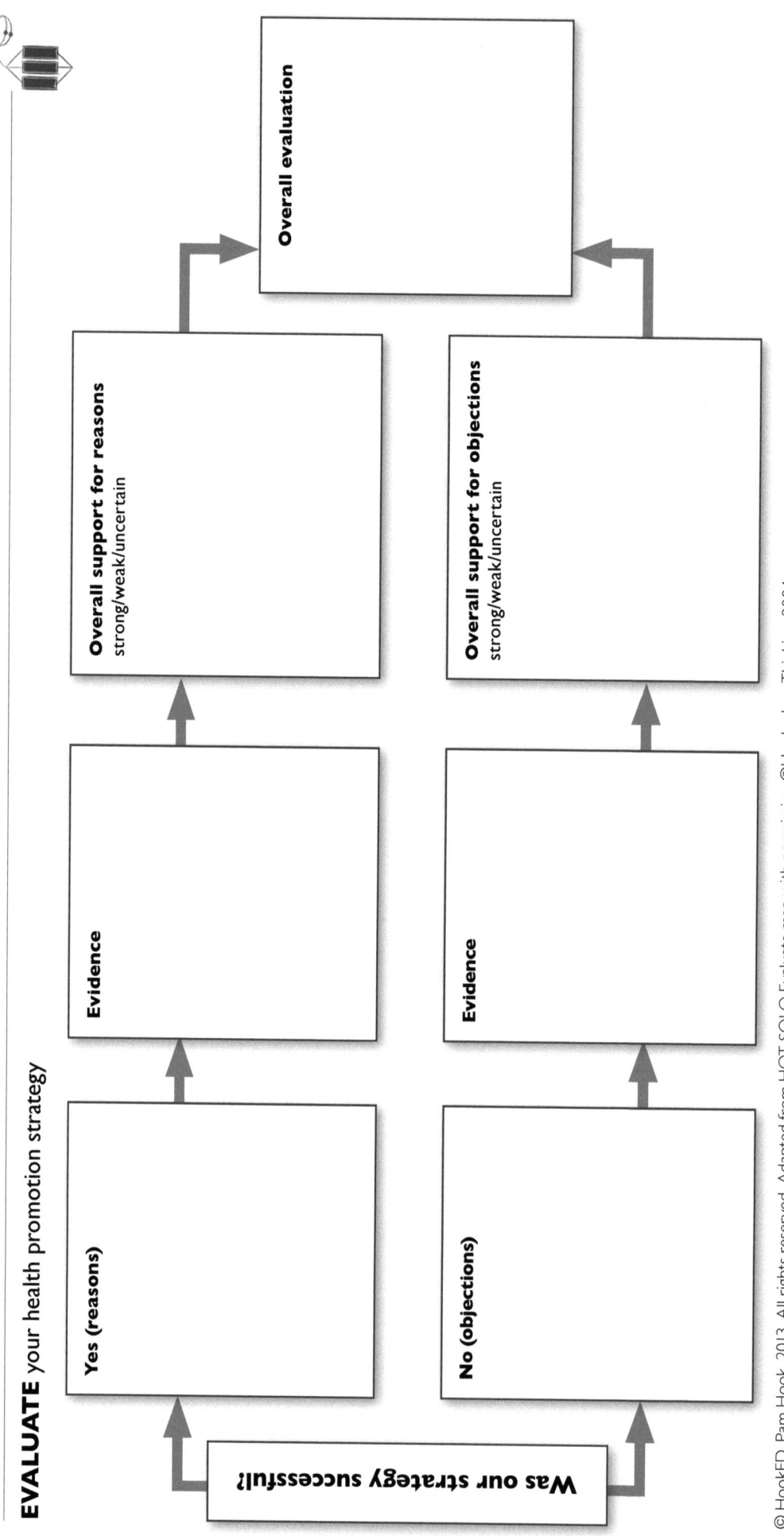

Table 3.4: HOT SOLO Evaluate rubric – health promotion strategy

SOLO level	Success criteria	Student exemplar
Extended abstract	**Visual map** **Text** … and it checks the reliability and validity of facts in the reasons and objections. It judges the reasons and objections individually and collectively and forms a generalisation.	… I believe the evidence supports holding Zumba classes to build wellbeing in communities. The evidence is strong that participants are fitter, have better balance and enjoy more social connections than they did before the classes. The few people who did not enjoy the activity are in a minority – they need a more specialised health promoting strategy and will be followed up so we can find a strategy to better meet their needs.
Relational	**Visual map** **Text** My evaluation identifies the argument and gives reasons for the argument and explains why these reasons support it (helping premise); and objections to the argument and explains why these objections work against it (helping premise) …	… This is because regular physical activity kept participants healthy, better balance protected them from injury and falls and the opportunity to make new friends made people feel needed. … So the classes did not build wellbeing for those who stopped coming – it possibly damaged their hearing temporarily and/or permanently and probably increased their feelings of isolation and depression. …
Multistructural	**Visual map** **Text** My evaluation identifies the argument and gives reasons for *and* objections to the argument.	My Zumba classes helped wellbeing in the community by building fitness, enhancing balance and agility, and encouraging new friendships. … However, some participants said the music was too loud and felt they were being judged on their body size – they stopped coming after the first session. …
Unistructural	**Visual map** **Text** My evaluation identifies the argument and gives reasons for *or* objections to the argument.	My Zumba classes helped wellbeing in the community by building participant fitness.
Prestructural	**Visual map** **Text** I need help to make an evaluation.	I do not know if my health promotion Zumba activity class made any difference to the people involved.

© HookED, Pam Hook, 2013. All rights reserved. Adapted from HOT SOLO Evaluate rubric with permission ©Hooked on Thinking, 2004.

4. Planning a student workbook with constructive alignment

I can see how to get to the next level for a physical skill with a SOLO rubric.

Year 9 PE student

Planning a student workbook that develops, connects and extends student learning in PE is made easier with backward design and SOLO. In this process, teachers:

- clearly identify the big picture – and associated achievement objectives and intended learning outcomes
- develop learning intentions and success criteria to reach the big picture outcomes
- design learning activities and resources to meet these criteria (the constructive alignment process of Biggs and Tang 2007).

PE students build deep understanding when their workbook learning experiences are scaffolded in this way – when educators provide more than activities that involve filling in the gaps, labelling diagrams and matching items. When teachers use SOLO learning verbs and constructive alignment to differentiate learning tasks across the SOLO levels of learning outcomes, then in our experience, both expectations and outcomes are enhanced.

The constructive alignment app on the HookED website (http://pamhook.com/solo-apps/learning-intention-generator) supports PE teachers wanting to plan in this way.

Seven-step planning process

Below is one possible approach to planning and designing a student workbook. It is followed by an example of a student workbook that resulted from this process.

Step 1: What is the big idea – the concept?

In this first step, identify big picture learning goals relevant to the essence of the PE curriculum. These goals should be relevant to developing the wellbeing of students and able to be achieved through movement contexts.

The evidence-based behaviours that lead to improvements in mental health and wellbeing are well established: connect, be active, take notice, keep learning and give (Thompson and Aked 2011). These five public health messages, developed by the new economics foundation (nef), form part of the UK government's Foresight Project on Mental Capital and Wellbeing.

"Be active" is a big idea of relevance to Year 9 students. Thompson and Aked (2011) describe it in this way:

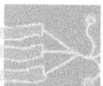

Go for a walk or run. Step outside. Cycle. Play a game. Garden. Dance. Exercising makes you feel good. Most importantly, discover a physical activity you enjoy and that suits your level of mobility and fitness.

This idea is useful to students now, given they can adopt more sedentary lifestyles through adolescence and early adulthood. It is also likely to remain relevant in the future when they will be living in a rapidly changing world where being tethered to a screen may reduce the need and the opportunities for physical activity.

Step 2: Find a context

Set learning goals in the Year 9 workbook that explore the big ideas to do with "be active" and the role these ideas play in wellbeing in local and community contexts, values and key competencies. This approach makes the goals relevant to students by introducing different perspectives from families, whānau and community and encouraging students to extend their understanding.

For example, learning goals in the workbook may include opportunities to:
- develop and improve being active at school and in the local community, based on the local context
- develop "being active" through values of community and participation
- identify ways in which students can practise the key competencies of managing self and participating and contributing (see Table 4.1).

Table 4.1: Examples of contexts that learning goals may incorporate

Context	New Zealand Curriculum values	New Zealand Curriculum key competencies
Being active in school sport and/or my local community	Excellence, innovation, diversity, equity, **community and participation**, ecological sustainability, integrity, respect	Thinking, **managing self, participating and contributing**, relating to others, making meaning from language symbols and text

Step 3: Make explicit links to the New Zealand Curriculum

In this step, make explicit links to the relevant learning area and achievement objectives of the New Zealand Curriculum (see Table 4.2).

Table 4.2: Example of planning with links to the curriculum

Health and physical education
Strand: Personal health and physical development **Focus:** Regular physical activity **Achievement objective:** Demonstrate an increasing sense of responsibility for incorporating regular and enjoyable physical activity into their personal lifestyle to enhance wellbeing. (Level 4)
Strand: Movement concepts and motor skills **Focus:** Science and technology **Achievement objective:** Investigate and experience ways in which scientific, technological and environmental knowledge and resources assist in and influence people's participation in regular physical activity. (Level 5)
Strand: Healthy communities and environments **Focus:** Community resources **Achievement objective:** Investigate and access a range of community resources that support wellbeing and evaluate the contribution made by each to the wellbeing of community members. (Level 4)

Source: Curriculum information drawn from Ministry of Education (2007)

Step 4: Generate differentiated learning intentions

Use constructive alignment and SOLO learning verbs to generate differentiated learning intentions. Table 4.3 offers an example of possible differentiated learning intentions for one of the achievement objectives identified in the previous example (Table 4.2 above).

Table 4.3: Example of differentiated learning intentions

Developed with constructive alignment and SOLO learning verbs

Achievement objective: Investigate and experience ways in which scientific, technological and environmental knowledge and resources assist in and influence people's participation in regular physical activity [exercise]. (Level 5) (Ministry of Education 2007)

Learning intentions		
Multistructural	**Relational**	**Extended abstract**
• Experience regular physical activity. • Observe physical activity occurring regularly in a named location over a given time. • List the physical activities occurring regularly in a named location over a given time. • Define regular physical activity. • Describe a physical activity occurring regularly in a named location over a given time. • Describe aspects of fitness. • Identify opportunities to be physically active in your local community. • Describe opportunities to be physically active in your local community. • Mark out a favourite physical activity route in your local area using the Map Maker function on Google Maps (under Tools). • Identify different fitness apps on smart phones (eg, NIKE fit club, runkeeper). • Describe different fitness apps on smart phones (eg, NIKE fit club, runkeeper). • Assess and monitor your personal level of physical activity (eg, use a fitness app to track your level of physical activity).	• Classify the physical activities occurring regularly in a named location over a given time. • Sequence the steps in a physical activity occurring regularly in a named location. • Sequence the physical activities occurring regularly in a named location over a given time. • Compare and contrast two different physical activities occurring in a named location over a given time. • Explain the causes for a physical activity occurring regularly in a named location over a given time. • Explain the effects of a physical activity occurring regularly in a named location over a given time. • Interview a participant in a physical activity occurring regularly in a named location over a given time. • Annotate a favourite walking route in your local area, choosing explanations for the route using the Map Maker function on Google Maps. • Explain the reasons for and effects of a fitness app. • Compare and contrast two different fitness apps.	• Reflect on any changes in your own regular physical activity as a result of this unit. • Reflect on any changes in your own understanding of the role of regular physical activity in wellbeing as a result of this unit. • Evaluate the ease of use of a fitness app. • Evaluate how much the use of the fitness app has contributed to the wellbeing of yourself and your local community. • Collaborate with others to create a physical activity route map that will engage people in your local area, for example, by using the Map Maker function on Google Maps. • Invite family and people in your community to have regular physical activity through a weekly route map challenge. • Build an online and offline community with local people by encouraging route map participants to add to your online map with engaging placemarks, descriptions or challenges, alternative route lines, photos and video. Optional: Integrate different fitness app readings into your challenge. • Evaluate how much your mapping initiative has assisted you and others to participate in regular physical activity.

Step 5: Develop learning experiences to create a student workbook

Elaborate on the relevant differentiated learning intentions to produce learning activities and experiences for students. Choose the most appropriate learning intentions to meet the learning needs of the students and the community involved. Integrate SOLO process maps and self assessment rubrics as writing frames where appropriate (for an example, see the workbook at the end of this section).

Step 6: Create SOLO-differentiated self assessment rubrics

For formative assessment of student progress, create SOLO-differentiated rubrics that students can use to assess their progress through the unit for:

- functioning knowledge outcomes – see Table 4.4 for an example
- declarative knowledge outcomes – see Table 4.5 for an example.

Table 4.4: How am I going (functioning knowledge)?

Use this rubric to assess progress in your functioning knowledge as we go through the unit

Concept: "Be active" for wellbeing	Context		
	Regular physical activity (exercise) for wellbeing (personal and community)	**Community resources** used for regular physical activity (exercise) – wellbeing	**Technology** used to support regular physical activity (exercise) – wellbeing
Prestructural	I need help to demonstrate any regular physical activity.	I need help to use community resources for regular physical activities.	I need help to use technology to support regular physical activity – wellbeing.
Unistructural	My life involves regular physical activity if prompted by others.	I use community resources for regular physical activity if prompted or directed.	I use technology to support regular physical activity – wellbeing – if I am prompted or directed.
Multistructural	My life usually involves some form of regular physical activity. But sometimes I really cannot be bothered.	I use community resources for regular physical activity …	I use technology to support regular physical activity – wellbeing …
Relational	My life usually involves some form of regular physical activity and I can justify why this activity is worth the effort each day …	… and I can justify why using community resources enhances my wellbeing …	… and I can justify why the use of technology supports regular physical activity …
Extended abstract	… and I seek feedback on how I can improve this physical activity to enhance my wellbeing … and I take action to support others seeking ways to introduce regular physical activity into their lives.	… and I can take action to support others using community resources to introduce regular physical activity into their lives.	… and I can take action to support others using technology to introduce regular physical activity into their lives.

© Essential Resources Educational Publishers Ltd, 2013

Table 4.5: How am I going (declarative knowledge)?

Use this rubric to assess progress in your declarative knowledge as we go through the unit

Concept: "Be active" for wellbeing	Contexts		
	Regular physical activity (exercise) for wellbeing (personal and community)	**Community resources** used for regular physical activity (exercise) – wellbeing	**Technology** used to support regular physical activity (exercise) – wellbeing
Prestructural	I need help to understand regular physical activity and wellbeing.	I need help to understand community resources for regular physical activity – wellbeing.	I need help to understand technology used for regular physical activity – wellbeing.
Unistructural	I can tell you: one relevant idea about fitness and wellbeing; one effect of exercise on wellbeing; and one component of fitness for a named sport.	I can find one place to exercise in my community.	I can tell you what my fitness test results were.
Multistructural	I can describe many aspects of fitness and wellbeing … I can describe many effects of exercise on wellbeing … I can state several components of fitness for a given sport …	I can find and describe a range of places to exercise in my community …	I can elaborate on what my fitness test results mean …
Relational	… and connect these aspects to wellbeing … and explain why the effects are important … and compare and contrast the fitness components for a range of sports …	… and compare and contrast the different places …	… and make connections between the fitness test results, my sports and my wellbeing …
Extended abstract	… and evaluate my own response to exercise … and create goals to improve aspects of fitness.	… and evaluate the best place for me to exercise.	… and create a fitness profile for a specific sport.

Step 7: Provide extension and challenge for students

Plan for independent inquiry and research to extend and challenge students who are successful in the supported inquiry using SOLO maps. Tasker's seven-step action competence learning model (Tasker 2000, cited in Robertson 2005) is another pedagogical approach to student inquiry that PE teachers use.

Tasker's stages are useful for fostering critical thinking and action when exploring physical activity from individual and social perspectives. Furthermore students are still able to use SOLO Taxonomy to self assess their level of competency at any stage of the action competence process (see Table 4.6).

Table 4.6: SOLO functioning knowledge rubric for outcomes

Developed using Tasker's action competence process

SOLO level	Level of competence	Effective strategies, including strategies from students
Prestructural	I have no idea how to [insert element]* in PE.	Show them examples. Demonstrate. Provide opportunity to practise.
Unistructural	I can [insert element]* in PE if I am reminded or prompted.	Clear instructions (step-by-step). Prompt. Do situational teaching.
Multistructural	I can [insert element]* in PE …	Revisit, recap and remind.
Relational	… and make links between [what I do] and a successful PE lesson … [justify]	Give repeated opportunities to practise and think about connections.
Extended abstract	… and I can evaluate my ability to [insert element]* in PE … and/or assist others to make good decisions in relation to [insert element]* in PE … and/or create a set of guidelines for [insert element]* in PE … and/or apply [insert element]* outside the PE lesson.	

Note: * Elements come from Tasker's action competence process. The following are examples:

- Identify an issue of relevance to community wellbeing.
- Engage in critical thinking process to develop in-depth knowledge about this issue.
- Think creatively to develop a vision with respect to the issue.
- Gather information, and analyse and evaluate it to gain a deeper understanding of the issue and what can be done to address it.
- Make an action plan to address the issue, identifying both barriers and enablers.
- Take action to complete the tasks assigned in step 5.
- Critically reflect on and evaluate their planning and acting.

Example of a student workbook

The following workbook example for Years 9–10 comes from the PE department at St Andrew's College in Christchurch. Setting it in context, in the box below, Struan George reflects on the experience of working with the SOLO resources in the workbook at the college. This workbook was developed using the planning process set out in the first part of this section.

> **Review of fitness studies – a SOLO approach to resources**
>
> As part of our "Sharpen Up" unit in Year 10 health and physical education, we look at fitness, components of fitness and how we can go about improving personal fitness. This year I was fortunate enough to use the "Fitness Studies – A SOLO Approach" resources with my class.
>
> The structure of the resources fitted easily into our current unit and the resources complemented (and in places replaced) current worksheets. The thing I found most useful about the resources was the "How am I going?" rubric. This provided an excellent reference point for students to monitor their personal progress through the unit. With the use of learning logs, students were easily able to identify where they were (feedback) and where to next (feed forward). This was performed using both self and peer assessment. Through the use of the rubric, students had a clear understanding of what they were learning and what was taught in the unit.
>
> In reference to the SOLO maps, I also found these very useful. The resource had great transition between maps and again the students found they understood the direction the unit was heading.
>
> Of particular note was the use of the "hexagons" activity. This created excellent discussion amongst groups and at a class level. This was quite an adaptable resource as students could "prioritise" a hierarchy of components for sports, and then compare and contrast between different sports. It was a great activity to generate student discussion and increased learner engagement through prolonged concentration and focus towards the learning tasks.
>
> Overall I feel that this is a wonderful resource for the ease in which we were able to use the resource to complement our existing programme and to further engage our students in the learning process. I would strongly recommend this resource to all physical educators!
>
> Struan George
> Physical education and health teacher
> St Andrews College
> Christchurch
> New Zealand

Fitness Studies – A SOLO Approach

Big idea

What is fitness?? Why do we need to be fit? How do we get fit? Where can we get fit? This unit looks at how fitness plays a role in wellbeing and the opportunities in our community to develop and improve fitness. It uses SOLO Taxonomy to encourage you to think deeply and make connections in your learning.

Key objectives

- Demonstrate an increasing sense of responsibility for incorporating regular and enjoyable physical activity into their personal lifestyle to enhance wellbeing. (Level 4)
- Investigate and access a range of community resources that support wellbeing and evaluate the contribution made by each to the wellbeing of community members. (Level 4)
- Investigate and experience ways in which scientific, technological and environmental knowledge and resources assist in and influence people's participation in regular physical activity. (Level 5)

How to use this workbook

Make sure you have this for every lesson, and complete the activities as your teacher tells you. Some activities with be in class while others may need to be done out of class either before or after a lesson. Keep it neat and tidy and do your best thinking!!

How am I going?

Use this rubric to assess your progress as you go through the unit.

I know nothing about fitness or exercise.	I can tell you one effect of exercise on wellbeing.	I can describe a range of effects of exercise on wellbeing …	… and make connections between the effects …	… and evaluate my own response to exercise.
	I can tell you one thing about fitness.	I can describe many aspects of fitness …	… and explain why they are important …	… and create plans to improve aspects of fitness.
	I can tell you what my fitness test results were.	I can tell you what my fitness test results were …	… and connect the results to my sports and wellbeing.	
	I can tell you one relevant component of fitness for a sport.	I can tell you the relevant components of fitness for a particular sport.	I can compare and contrast the relevant components of fitness for a range of sports …	… and create a fitness profile for a specific sport.
	I can find one place to exercise in my community.	I can find and describe a range of places to exercise in my community …	… and compare and contrast the different places …	… and evaluate the best place for me to exercise.
(KC) I cannot motivate myself to try my best in every lesson.	I will try my best in lessons if I'm reminded.	I am motivated to try my best in every lesson …	… and can see the impact it has on my performance and the lesson …	… and can apply it in other settings / be a role model.

So ... what is fitness??

Use this page to create a definition of fitness. **Think** and put your own ideas on the map, then get into a **pair** and talk through your ideas and then **share** your ideas with the class to get a range of viewpoints. Finally collate the ideas into a definition and write it into the box at the bottom.

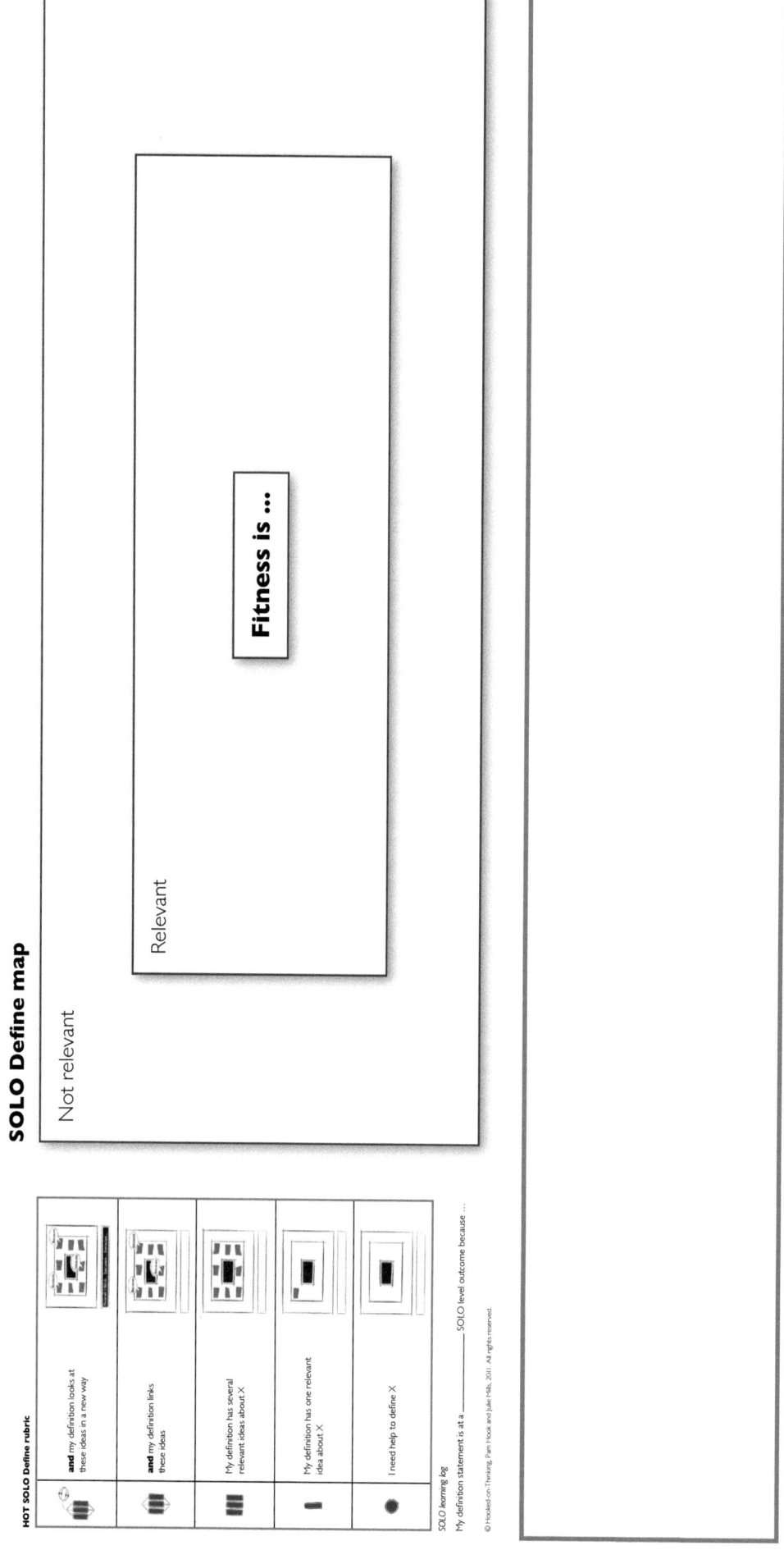

And ... what are the good things about exercise?
Use a SOLO Describe+ map to record your thinking.

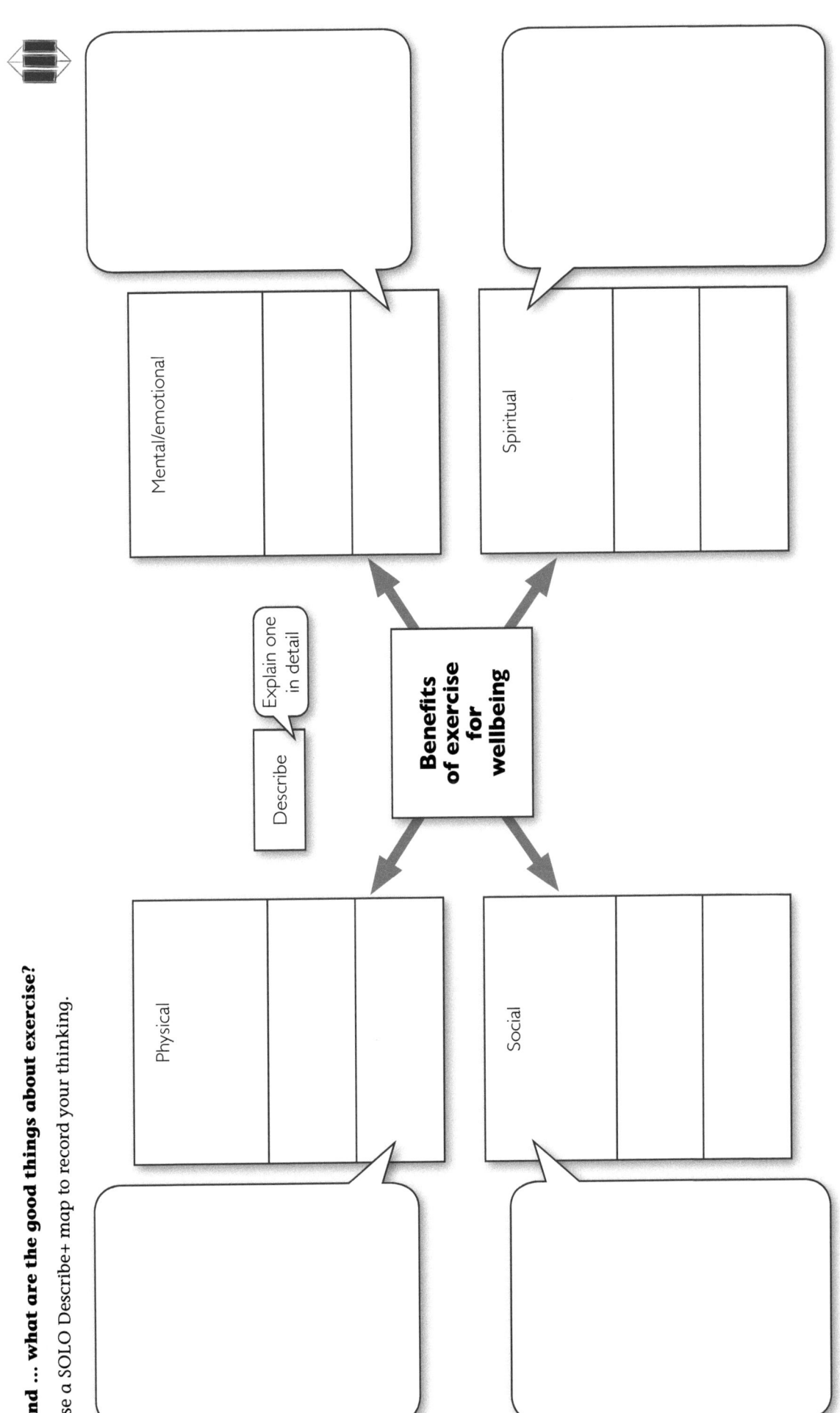

Now ... let's look at fitness in more detail

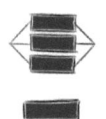

There are many different components of fitness and they can be **classified** into two categories. Decide which component of fitness goes in which category and using your own knowledge and what you have been doing in class write a brief **definition** for each one. Use a SOLO Classify map to record your thinking.

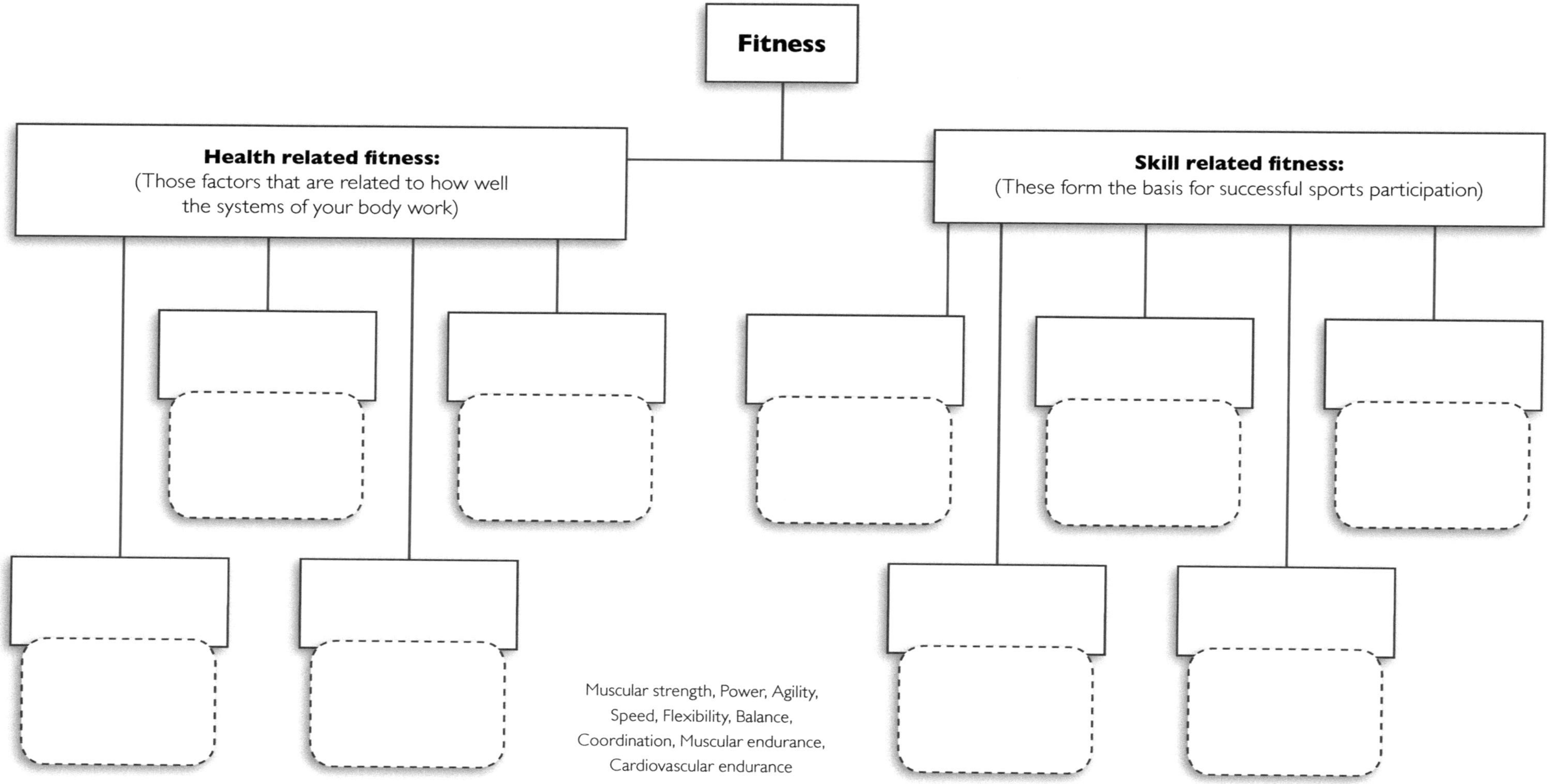

Fitness

Health related fitness:
(Those factors that are related to how well the systems of your body work)

Skill related fitness:
(These form the basis for successful sports participation)

Muscular strength, Power, Agility, Speed, Flexibility, Balance, Coordination, Muscular endurance, Cardiovascular endurance

Fitness components and sport

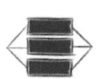

Cut out the hexagons and arrange them in different ways to show the links between sports and the fitness components. You can add your own sports in the blank hexagons.

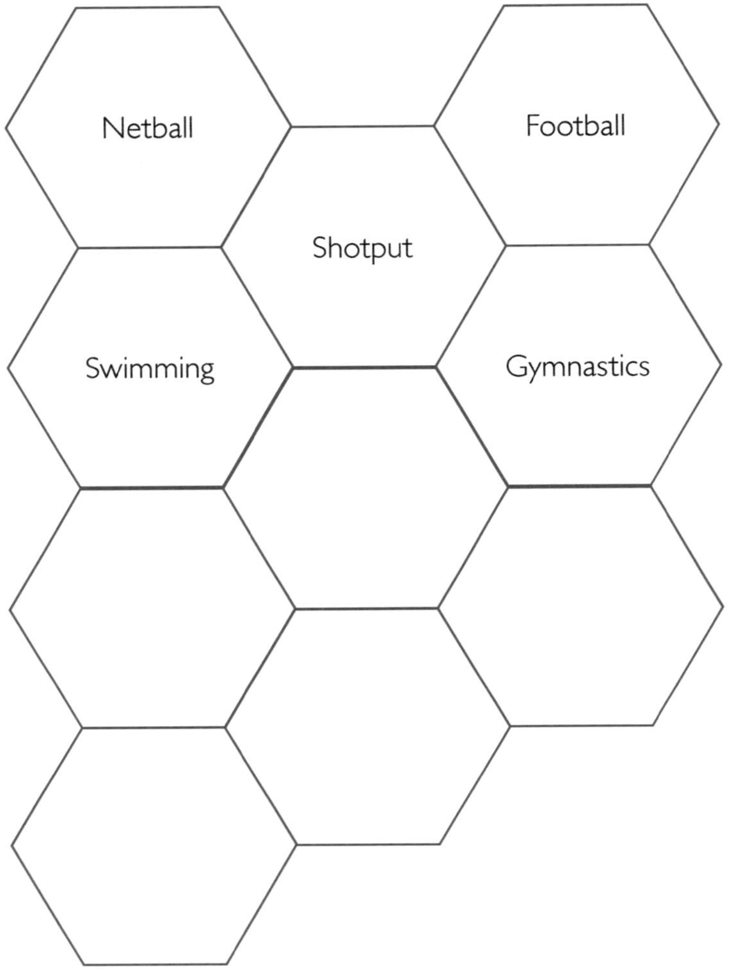

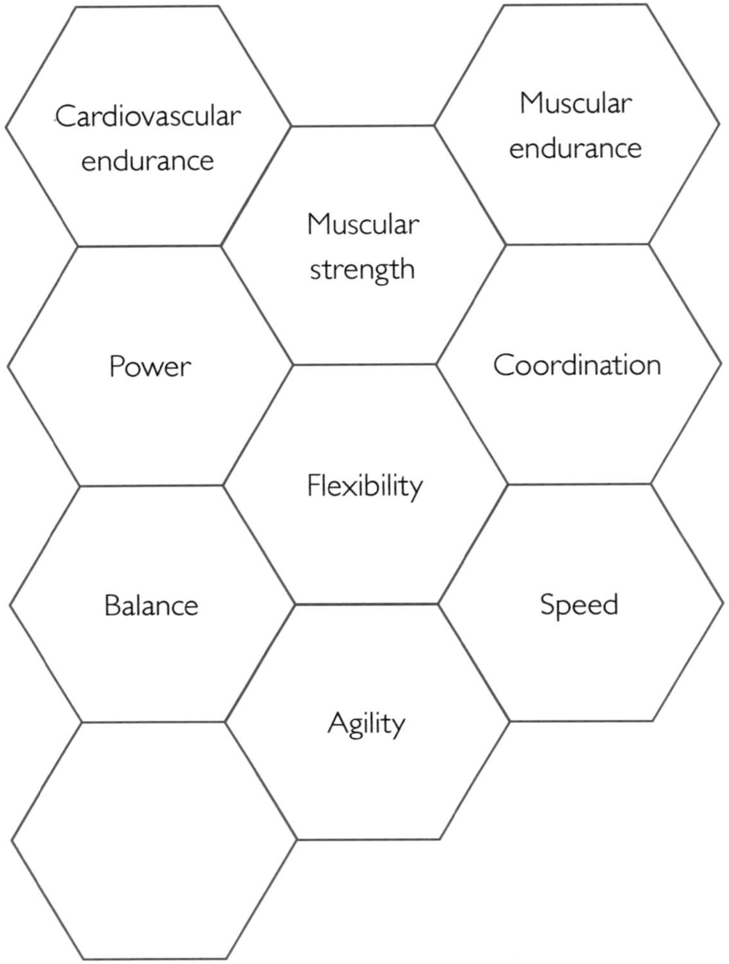

Sports hexagons: Football, Gymnastics, Shotput, Netball, Swimming (plus blank hexagons)

Fitness components hexagons: Muscular endurance, Coordination, Speed, Muscular strength, Flexibility, Agility, Cardiovascular endurance, Power, Balance

© Essential Resources Educational Publishers Ltd, 2013

Fitness components and sport (continued)

Choose two sports or physical activities and **compare** and **contrast** the fitness components involved. Use a SOLO Compare and Contrast map to record your thinking.

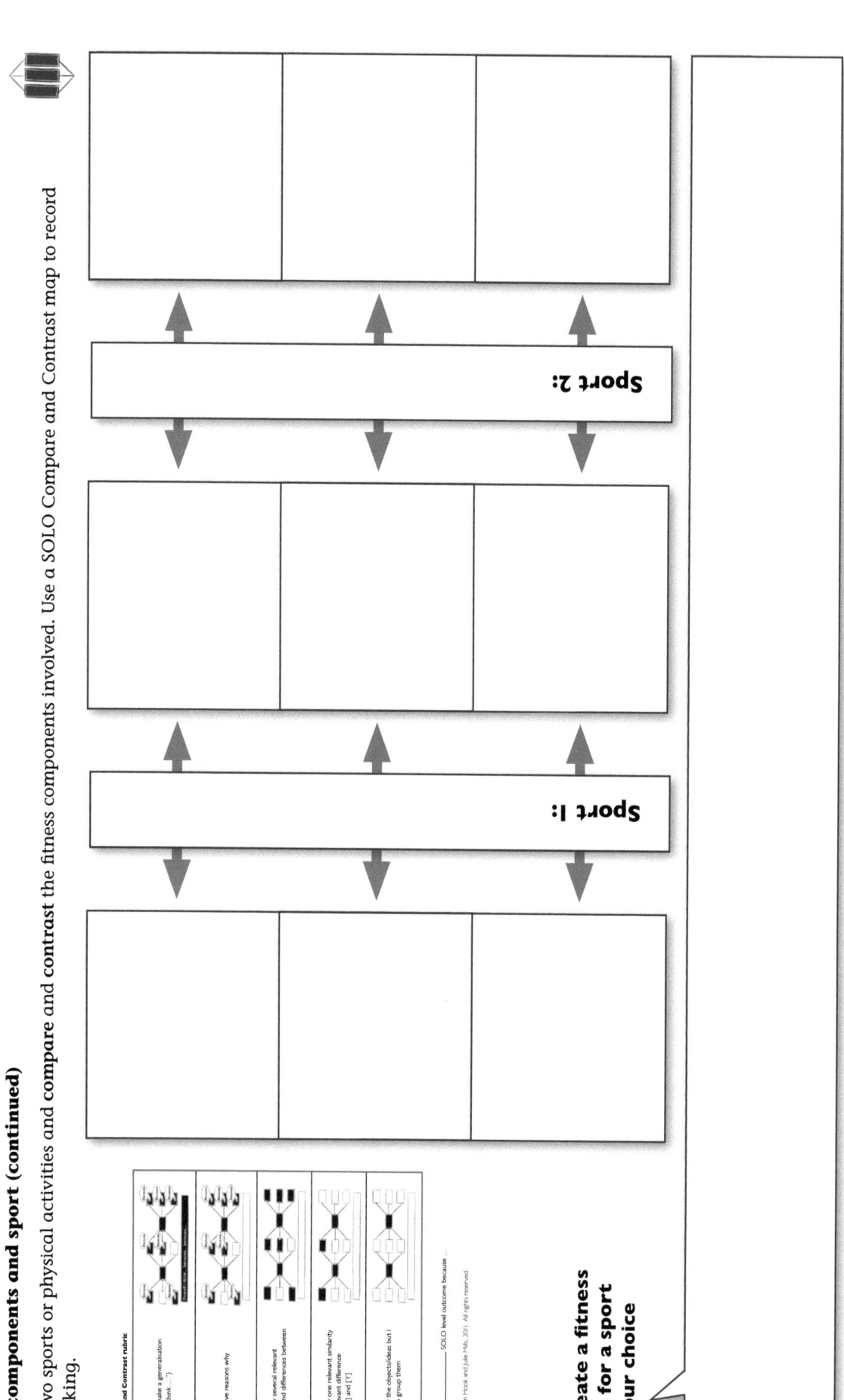

My fitness results

Use the SOLO paragraph structure to connect ideas about your fitness results.

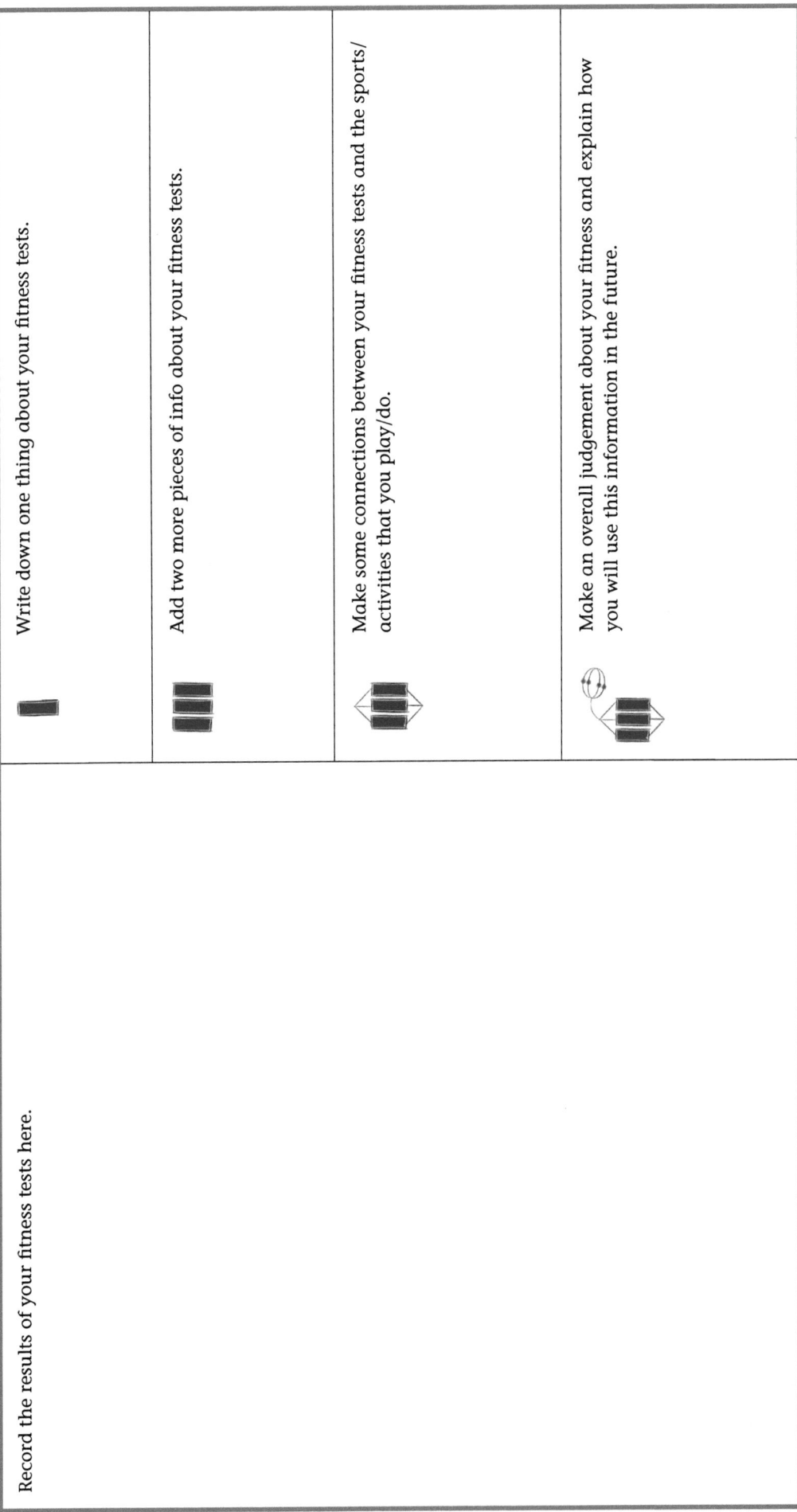

Record the results of your fitness tests here.

Write down one thing about your fitness tests.

Add two more pieces of info about your fitness tests.

Make some connections between your fitness tests and the sports/activities that you play/do.

Make an overall judgement about your fitness and explain how you will use this information in the future.

Ways to improve my fitness

As you try out different ways of improving your fitness in class, fill out this SOLO Describe++ map.

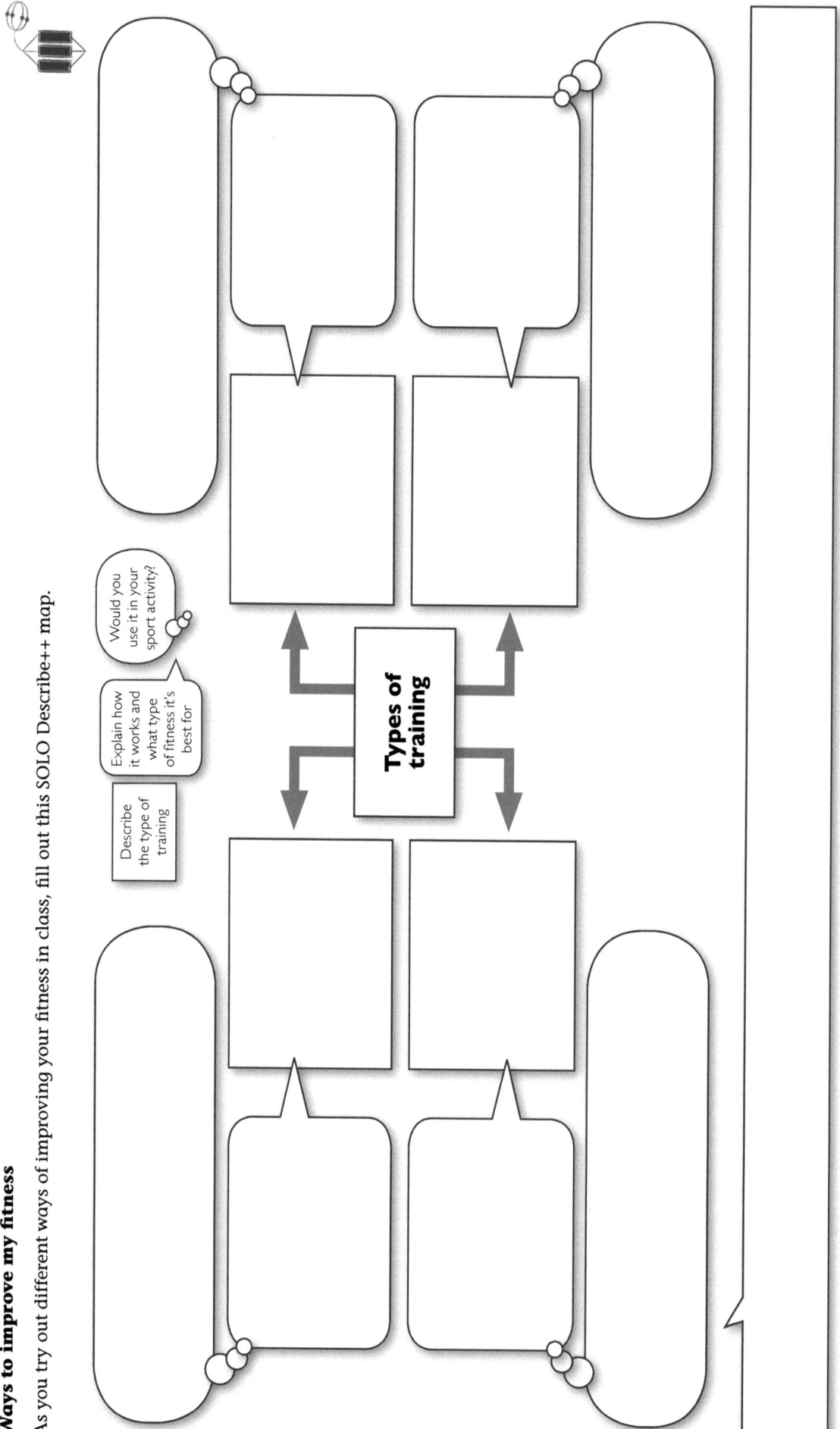

Describe the type of training

Explain how it works and what type of fitness it's best for

Would you use it in your sport activity?

Types of training

Technology and fitness

Use this SOLO Cause and Effect map to explain the impact of different smart phone apps on individual training.

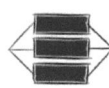

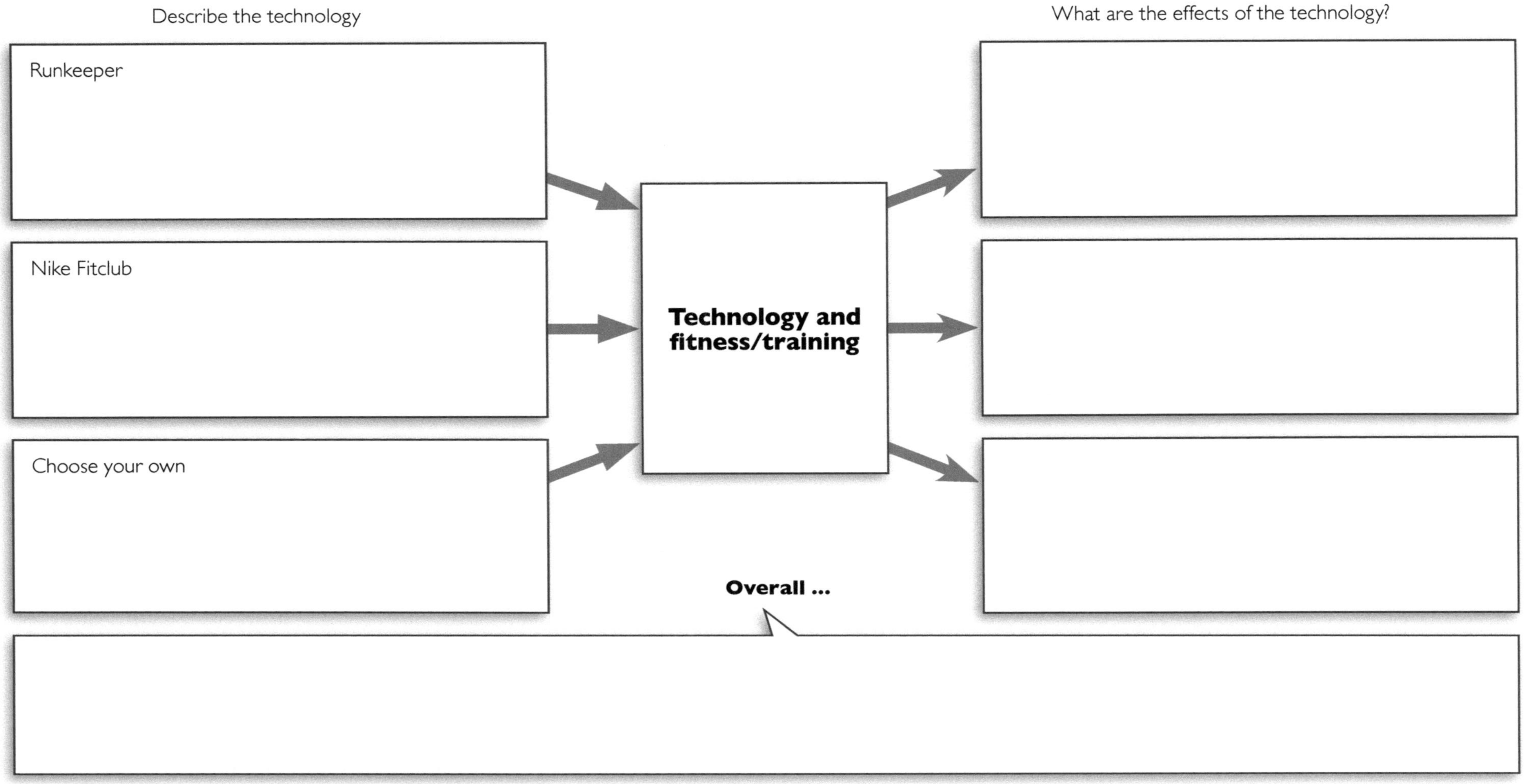

Describe the technology

What are the effects of the technology?

- Runkeeper
- Nike Fitclub
- Choose your own

Technology and fitness/training

Overall …

Where can I get fit? A home learning task

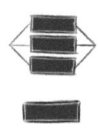

Part 1: Find a map of your local area on the internet, print it and identify the places on the map where you can exercise.

Part 2: Choose 4 of the facilities from Part 1 and complete the SOLO Describe++ map to decide which one is the best for you (highlight the best facility).

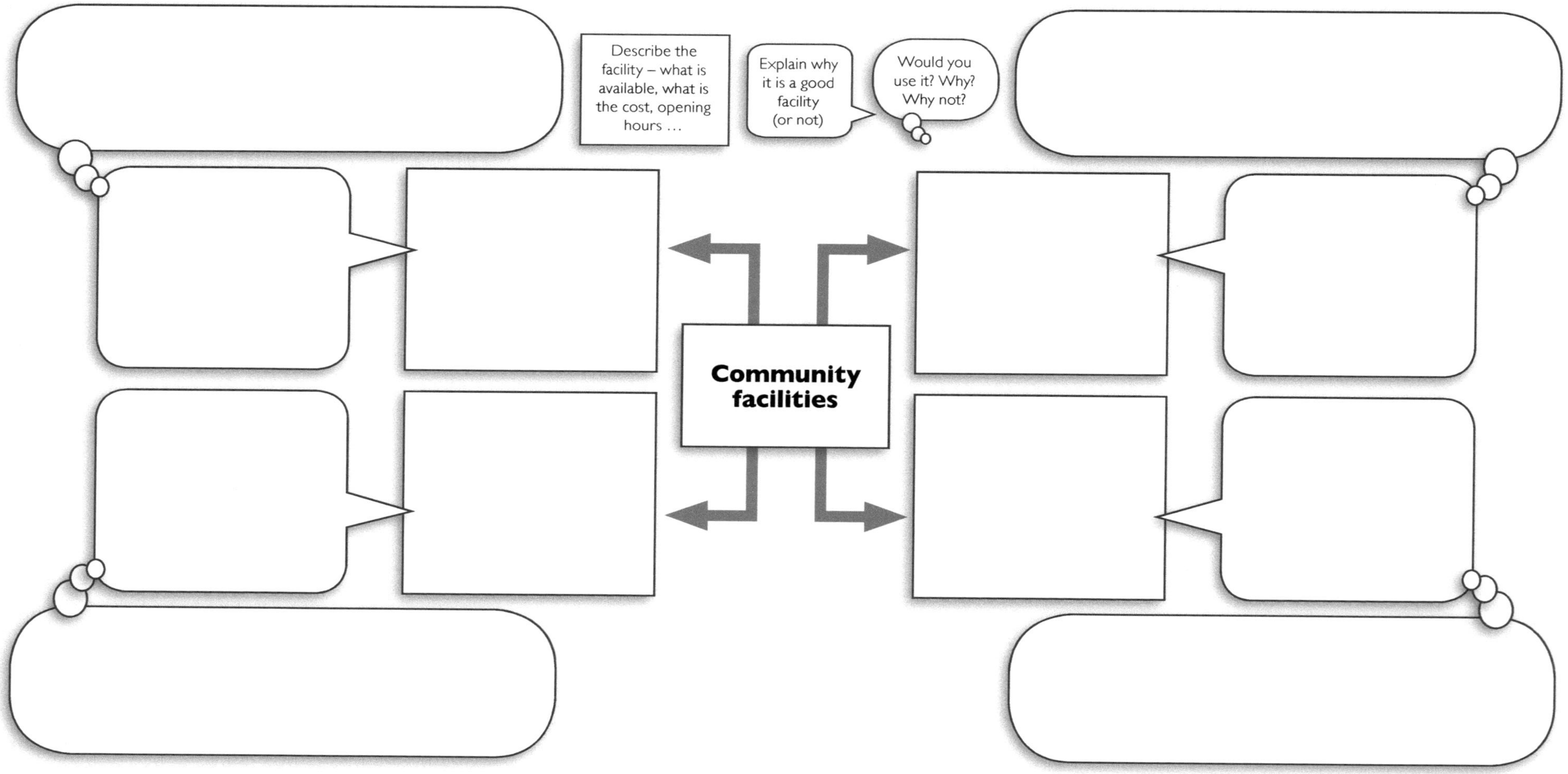

Community facilities

Describe the facility – what is available, what is the cost, opening hours ….

Explain why it is a good facility (or not)

Would you use it? Why? Why not?

Putting it all together

Use all of the information to create an action plan to improve a component of your fitness. Include:

- the component of fitness you would like to improve and why
- how you can test this component
- the type of training you are going to use and why
- where/when you would do your training and why
- what technology you could use
- how you will know if you have improved.

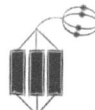

●	I	III	III	III
I do not know how to create an action plan.	I can create a simple action plan if someone helps me.	I can use a range of information to create a simple action plan.	I can link information to create a detailed action plan …	… and I can evaluate the success of the plan or apply the action plan outside PE.

Examples of completed SOLO maps with a fitness focus

Figures 4.1 to 4.3 illustrate some ways in which students have used SOLO Compare and Contrast, Classify and Describe++ maps in an inquiry into fitness, wellbeing and sport.

Figure 4.1: Using SOLO Compare and Contrast map to find similarities and differences between the fitness components of netball and gymnastics

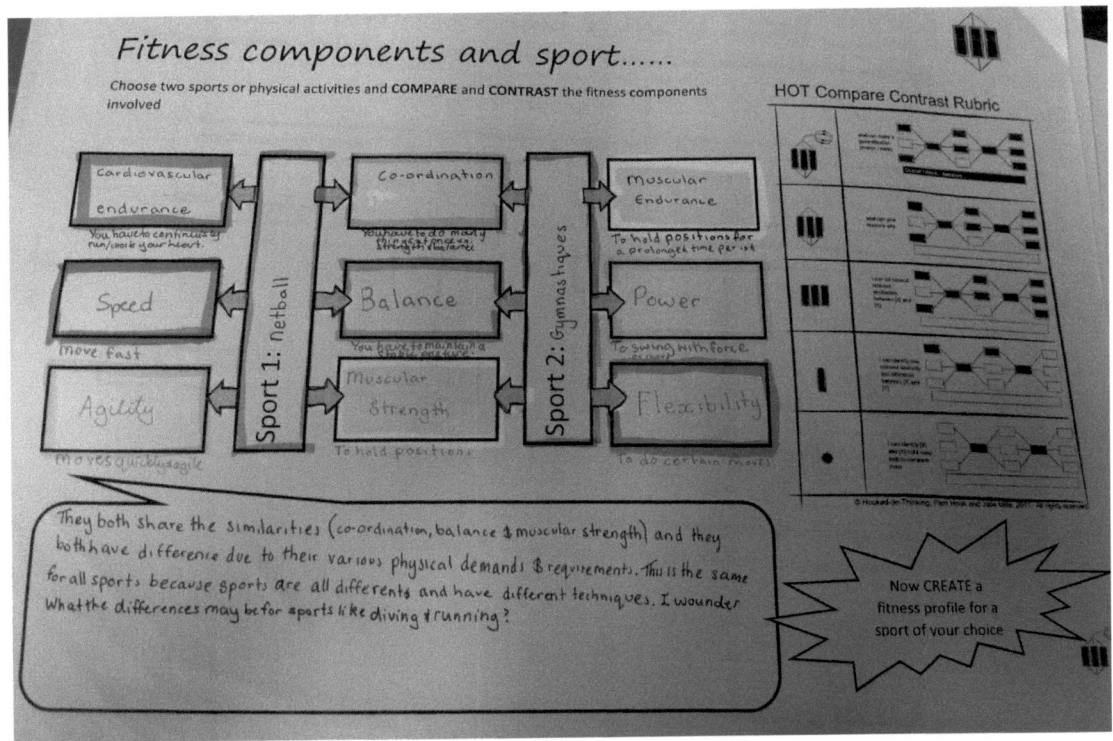

Figure 4.2: Using SOLO Classify map to categorise different components of fitness

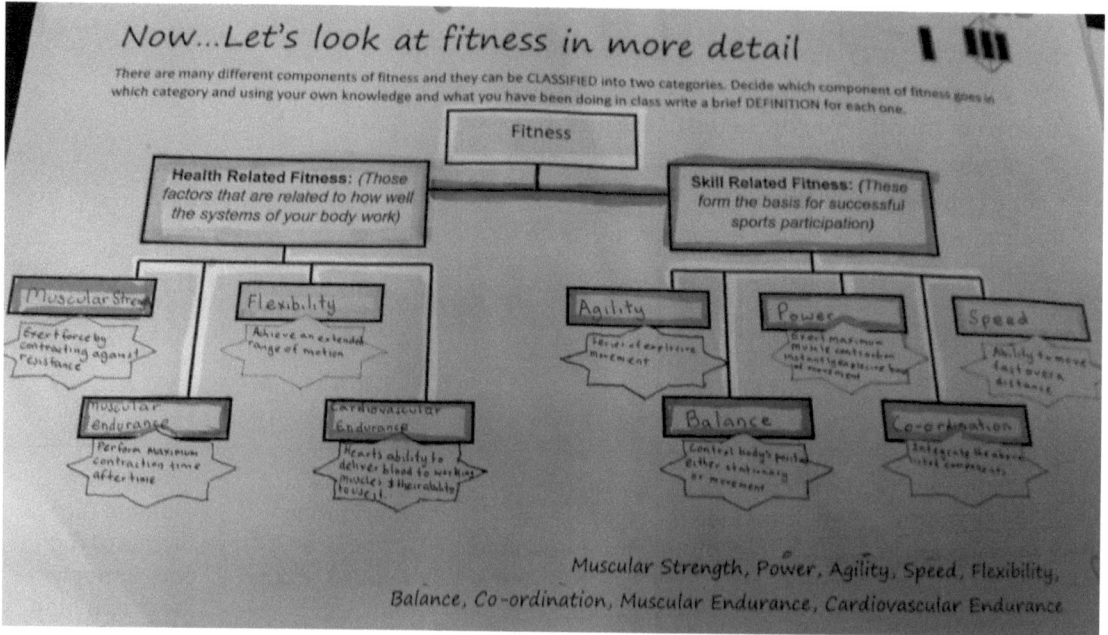

Figure 4.3: Using SOLO Describe++ map to describe, explain and evaluate community fitness facilities

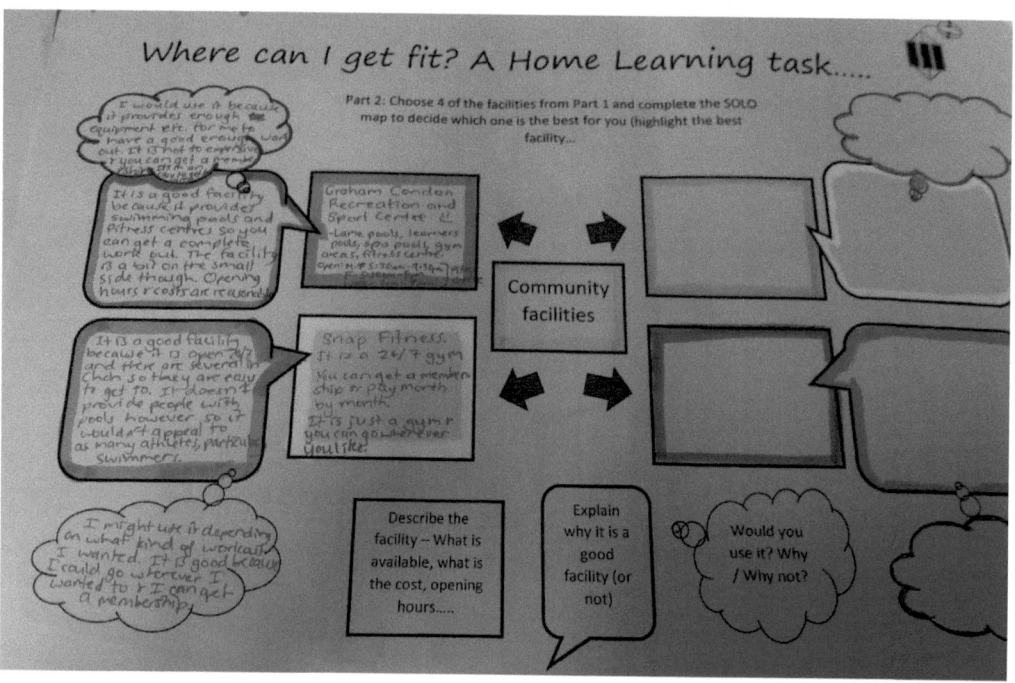

Conclusion

PE teachers work in gyms and pools, and on grass and turf, to provide students with learning experiences in movement contexts that help them develop the knowledge, skills, competencies, attitudes and behaviours needed for wellbeing. They face opportunities and challenges that differ from those faced by teachers whose pedagogies are mostly practised in classrooms.

Powerful strategies for making a difference to student achievement (Hattie 2012, pp 102–14) include:
- determining prior knowledge
- making links to students' previous experience
- designing learning experiences that bring in, and then connect and extend information and performance
- providing opportunities for metacognition and feedback (peer and teacher)
- giving students multiple ways to engage with an idea.

When PE teachers bring SOLO Taxonomy to these strategies they make learning visible (and thus accessible) for students. With SOLO as a model for learning outcomes, students and teachers can more easily determine the level of knowledge, skills, competencies and behaviours students bring to the lesson. They can more easily understand the complexity of the learning activity – as unistructural, multistructural, relational or extended abstract – and then students can self assess their progress using SOLO-differentiated success criteria. SOLO-differentiated assessment rubrics for functioning and declarative knowledge provide students with an explicit language for metacognition: What am I doing? How well is it going? What should I do next? Finally SOLO learning verbs provide teachers with multiple prompts for designing learning experiences that nudge up against the idea to be learnt in multiple ways.

When integrated into effective pedagogies for student achievement, SOLO is a powerful model for PE teachers wanting students to understand the depth and breadth of wellbeing through movement contexts. It allows students (and teachers) to distinguish between functioning and declarative knowledge; to demonstrate how physical activity can benefit academic achievement; to change the "What game are we playing today?" mind set that some Year 9 students bring to class; and to introduce and practise the key competencies and develop students' fluency in using them in their daily lives.

We have packed this series with practical examples and strategies showing how PE teachers might use SOLO as an effective pedagogy in junior secondary school. When PE students learn in, through and about movement experiences using SOLO, they not only develop physical and social skills – they have access to a model that fosters critical thinking and action for individual and social wellbeing.

References

Biggs, J and Collis, K. (1982). *Evaluating the Quality of Learning: The SOLO Taxonomy.* New York: Academic Press.

Biggs, J and Tang, C. (2007). *Teaching for Quality Learning at University. What the student does* (3rd ed). Berkshire: Society for Research into Higher Education & Open University Press.

Griffin, LL, Mitchell, SA and Oslin, JL. (1997). *Teaching Sport Concepts and Skills: A tactical games approach.* Champaign, IL: Human Kinetics.

Hattie, JAC. (2012). *Visible Learning for Teachers: Maximising impact on achievement.* Abingdon: Routledge.

Ministry of Education. (2007). *The New Zealand Curriculum: The English-medium teaching and learning in years 1–13.* Wellington: Learning Media.

Robertson, J. (2005). Making sense of health promotion in context of health and physical education curriculum learning. Paper commissioned by Ministry of Education for the Marautanga Curriculum Project.

Thompson, S and Aked. J. (2011). *Five Ways to Wellbeing: New applications, new ways of thinking.* London: nef. URL: www.neweconomics.org/publications/entry/five-ways-to-wellbeing (accessed 8 July 2013).

Werner, P. (1989). Teaching games: A tactical perspective. *Journal of Physical Education, Recreation and Dance,* 60(3), 97–101.

Printed by Libri Plureos GmbH in Hamburg, Germany